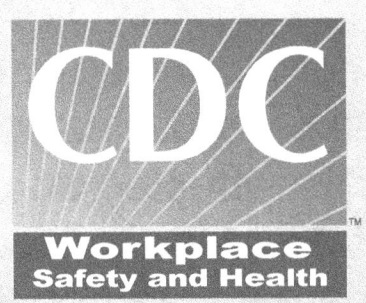

Workplace
Safety and Health

Exposures to Pharmaceutical Dust at a Mail Order Pharmacy – Illinois

Kenneth W. Fent, PhD
Srinivas Durgam, MSPH, MSChE, CIH
Carlos Aristeguieta, MD, MPH
Scott E. Brueck, MS, CIH

Health Hazard Evaluation Report
HETA 2010-0026-3150
December 2011

DEPARTMENT OF HEALTH AND HUMAN SERVICES
Centers for Disease Control and Prevention
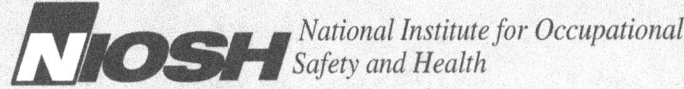
National Institute for Occupational
Safety and Health

The employer shall post a copy of this report for a period of 30 calendar days at or near the workplace(s) of affected employees. The employer shall take steps to insure that the posted determinations are not altered, defaced, or covered by other material during such period. [37 FR 23640, November 7, 1972, as amended at 45 FR 2653, January 14, 1980].

CONTENTS

ABBREVIATIONS

μg/m^3	Micrograms per cubic meter
μm	Micrometer
ACGIH®	American Conference of Governmental Industrial Hygienists
ADU	Automatic dispensing unit
AL	Action level
API	Active pharmaceutical ingredient
BVNA	Bureau Veritas North America, Inc.
CFR	Code of Federal Regulations
dB	Decibel
dBA	Decibels, A-scale
DESI/MS	Desorption electrospray ionization/mass spectrometry
HEPA	High-efficiency particulate air
HHE	Health hazard evaluation
HHPC	Handheld airborne particle counter
Hz	Hertz
IOM	Institute of Occupational Medicine
Lpm	Liters per minute
mL	Milliliter
mm	Millimeter
mg	Milligram
MDC	Minimum detectable concentration
MQC	Minimum quantifiable concentration
NA	Not applicable
NAICS	North American Industry Classification System
NIOSH	National Institute for Occupational Safety and Health
ND	None detected
OEL	Occupational exposure limit
OSHA	Occupational Safety and Health Administration
Particles/L	Particles per liter
PBZ	Personal breathing zone
PEL	Permissible exposure limit
PPE	Personal protective equipment
PTFE	Polytetrafluoroethylene
REL	Recommended exposure limit
STEL	Short-term exposure limit
TLV®	Threshold limit value
TWA	Time-weighted average
WEEL™	Workplace environmental exposure level

The National Institute for Occupational Safety and Health (NIOSH) received an employer request for a health hazard evaluation at a mail order pharmacy in Illinois concerning employee exposures to pharmaceutical dust and the potential health effects from these exposures. This request was later changed to include an evaluation of noise.

What NIOSH Did

- We visited the pharmacy in April 2010. We returned in December 2010 to do additional sampling.

- We measured particles over time at different processes. We did this to determine if pharmaceutical dust was released into the air.

- We sampled the air for dust. These air samples were weighed to determine the amount of dust in the air and analyzed for lactose (a common inactive ingredient) and active pharmaceutical ingredients (APIs).

- We measured noise levels in the pharmacy.

- We talked with employees privately about their symptoms and health concerns at work.

What NIOSH Found

- Dust was released into the air when cells were cleaned and canisters were filled with tablets.

- Lactose and APIs were found in the airborne dust. This suggests that some of the airborne dust was from pharmaceuticals.

- Levels of the two APIs we measured in air (warfarin and lisinopril) were below occupational exposure limits.

- Hazardous drugs were dispensed at the pharmacy. Some of these were tablets that could generate airborne dust. Hazardous drugs are drugs that are known or suspected to cause adverse health effects from exposures in the workplace.

- Surfaces in the pharmacy and employees' clothing could have pharmaceutical dust on them. This could lead to secondary exposure to employees and their families.

- A pharmacy technician working at the Baker machine had a noise exposure above NIOSH and Occupational Safety and Health Administration (OSHA) exposure limits of 85 A-weighted decibels. All other employees whom we monitored had noise exposures less than these exposure limits.

- Most of the noise came from the release of compressed air by pharmacy equipment.

- Some employees had eye and respiratory irritation.

What Managers Can Do

- Install tabletop ventilation booths for employees who hand fill hazardous drug prescriptions and for employees who clean, repair, and refill cells and canisters.

- Install movable capture hoods for employees who refill Baker machine canisters.

- Write procedures and establish a schedule for replacing the particulate filters in the ventilation booths and hoods. These procedures should list the required personal protective equipment.

- Identify and label all hazardous drugs.

- Modify the current procedure for hand filling hazardous drug prescriptions. These procedures should list all the personal protective equipment, control measures, and housekeeping practices needed to prevent exposures to employees.

- Require employees to wear NIOSH-approved half-mask N95-filtering facepiece respirators when hand filling hazardous drug prescriptions and changing out particulate filters in the ventilation booths, hoods, and HEPA vacuums. The use of respirators can be discontinued for hand filling of hazardous drug prescriptions when a ventilation booth is available for this process.

- Start a comprehensive respiratory protection program for employees who are required to wear respirators. This program should follow the OSHA respiratory protection standard.

- Provide employees with lab coats or other protective clothing that remains at the worksite. These items should be thrown away after each use or laundered weekly by professionals.

- Emphasize to employees the need to wear nitrile gloves when handling pharmaceuticals.

- Provide employees with easy access to hand washing stations. Employees should be required to wash their hands before eating, drinking, or using tobacco products.

- Install mufflers on the exhaust ports of solenoid valves and actuators.

- Fix any leaks in compressed air lines.

- Provide employees with hearing protection that has a noise reduction rating of 15–20 decibels. Pharmacy technicians working around the Baker machine should be required to wear this hearing protection.

- Do not allow employees to use personal music players because they can increase the risk of hearing loss.

- Create a health and safety committee. This committee should include employee and employer representatives who meet regularly to address health and safety concerns.

What Employees Can Do

- Follow the procedures for using and maintaining the ventilation booths and hoods.

- Follow all procedures when you fill a prescription for hazardous drugs.

- Wear gloves when handling pharmaceuticals.

- Wash your hands before you eat, drink, or use tobacco products.

- Tell your supervisor about any health or safety concerns you have.

- Wear hearing protection when you work near the Baker machine.

- Do not use personal music players.

- Become active in the health and safety committee.

Summary

NIOSH evaluated health symptoms, pharmaceutical dust, and noise exposures among employees at a mail order pharmacy. We found that dust was released, particularly during the cleaning, repairing, and refilling of cells and canisters. This dust contained APIs and lactose, a common ingredient in pharmaceuticals. Exposures to pharmaceutical dust could have contributed to eye and upper respiratory irritation reported by employees. High noise exposures were caused by release of compressed air, which could be reduced by installing noise controls.

NIOSH investigators conducted an HHE at a mail order pharmacy to determine whether employees were exposed to pharmaceutical dust and noise and were experiencing health effects related to these exposures. We observed work processes, practices, and workplace conditions. We collected air samples to characterize employees' exposures. We measured employees' noise exposures and sound levels in the production areas. We held confidential interviews with 45 employees to learn about their health and workplace concerns.

Using real-time particle meters, we identified releases of dust during the cleaning, repairing, and refilling of cells and canisters. We sampled the air for different sizes of dust particles and analyzed the samples for APIs and lactose, a common ingredient of pharmaceuticals. Most of these air samples contained lactose and one or more APIs, suggesting that some of the airborne dust came from pharmaceuticals. We quantified two APIs on these air samples, warfarin and lisinopril; the air concentrations were well below applicable OELs.

Most employees wore protective gloves but did not wear protective clothing when handling pharmaceuticals. Consequently, personal clothing could become contaminated with APIs and become a source of secondary exposure to employees or their family members. Many employees washed hands before eating or smoking, which should minimize the ingestion of APIs. Some employees voluntarily wore N95 filtering facepiece respirators. However, these respirators were not always worn or maintained correctly. Shortly before our second visit, pharmacy managers developed standard operating procedures for the handling of hazardous drugs. These procedures required hazardous drug prescriptions to be filled and verified in a separate area by dedicated personnel. Gloves were the only control measure required for this process.

The most likely health effects from exposure to APIs are allergic reactions and upper respiratory irritation. Nearly half the employees reported eye and upper respiratory irritation, which could be related to their exposures to APIs. However, these symptoms could also be caused by general dust exposures or non-occupational factors, such as weather conditions and seasonal allergies.

We were unable to quantify employees' exposures to all APIs. Given the uncertainty of our exposure assessment, the potential for surface and personal clothing contamination, and the lack of

SUMMARY
(CONTINUED)

knowledge regarding the toxicity of low-level exposures to multiple APIs, exposures to pharmaceutical dust should be reduced as much as feasible. We recommend installing ventilation booths and movable capture hoods that can be used when hand filling hazardous drug prescriptions and cleaning, repairing, and refilling cells and canisters. All hazardous drugs should be identified and labeled. All employees who handle drugs should wear lab coats or other protective clothing to minimize contamination of their personal clothing.

We found that full-shift TWA noise exposures for employees working near the Baker machines could exceed the OSHA AL and NIOSH REL of 85 dBA. Employees' noise exposures in other production areas were below these exposure limits. Some employees wore hearing protection, but the noise reduction rating was more than what was needed. We recommend providing hearing protectors with a noise reduction rating of 15–20 dB. We noted that many employees wore an earphone from a personal music player in one of their ears. Because this can increase the risk of hearing loss if the sound level from the earphone is higher than the background noise in the facility, we recommend that personal music players not be used in the workplace.

One-third octave band noise level measurements at several different work areas or around pharmacy equipment indicated that the highest noise levels occurred at high frequencies (greater than 8,000 Hz). To reduce noise levels and noise exposures, we recommend installing mufflers on the exhaust port of solenoid valves and actuators throughout the facility and constructing a better enclosure at the capper machine, located near the Baker machine.

Keywords: NAICS 446110 (Pharmacies and Drug Stores), drugs, pills, pill dust, active pharmaceutical ingredients, APIs, tablets, pharmaceuticals, mail order pharmacy, automatic pill dispensing machine, robotic pill dispenser, Hispanic, Spanish-speaking

This page left intentionally blank

INTRODUCTION

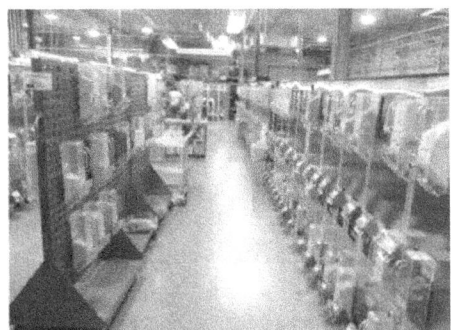

Figure 1. Platform above the Baker machine where canisters containing pharmaceuticals were loaded into the machine.

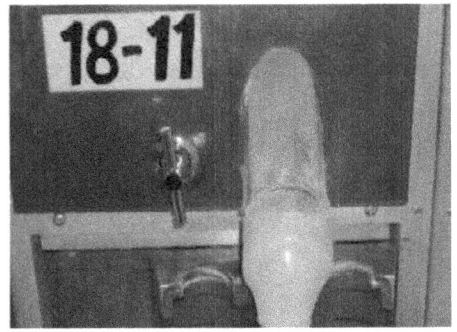

Figure 2. Baker machine nozzle where pharmaceuticals were dispensed into prescription bottles.

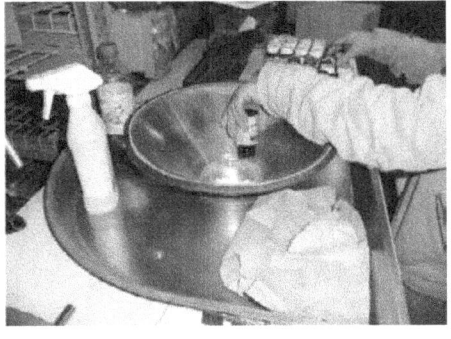

Figure 3. Employee in the offline replenishment area dumping tablets into a funnel that feeds into a Baker canister.

NIOSH received an HHE request from the management of a mail order pharmacy in Illinois concerning employee exposures to pharmaceutical dust and potential health effects from these exposures. In response to this HHE request, we conducted evaluations in April and December 2010. After our first visit, the pharmacy management asked us to evaluate noise exposures, which we did on the second visit.

The mail order pharmacy filled prescriptions using primarily automated distribution systems and delivered these prescriptions to its customers throughout the country. A total of 350 employees worked on the first or second shift. Spanish was the first language for a large percentage of the employees. The mail order pharmacy was divided into two areas: the pharmacy, where automatic dispensing machines were located and most prescriptions were filled, and the warehouse, where other activities were performed, such as manual counting and refilling of canisters. Two brands of automatic dispensing machines were used for high throughput prescriptions: Baker (one large customized machine, McKesson Corporation, San Francisco, California) and Optifill® (two smaller customized machines, AmerisourceBergen®, Valley Forge, Pennsylvania). Both machines used gravity to dispense pharmaceutical tablets and capsules.

The Baker machine had an elevated platform where the canisters containing pharmaceuticals were loaded into the machine (Figure 1). The pharmaceuticals were fed from a canister into a cell below the platform. A conveyor belt on the outside of the machine carried a prescription bottle to the nozzle below the appropriate cell (Figure 2), and a valve in the cell opened to dispense the pharmaceutical into the bottle. The Baker machine filled approximately 10,000 prescriptions per day during our evaluation. Two pharmacy technicians maintained the Baker machine. Their responsibilities included freeing jams, identifying bottles that did not receive pharmaceuticals, and cleaning and repairing malfunctioning cells. The Baker canisters were refilled in the offline replenishment area in the warehouse. In the offline replenishment area, two or three pharmacy technicians dumped bottles containing the appropriate pharmaceuticals into a funnel that fed into a labeled Baker canister (Figure 3).

Canisters were situated on the outside of each of the two Optifill machines (Figure 4). A conveyor belt carried prescription bottles through the middle of each machine. A bottle stopped below one

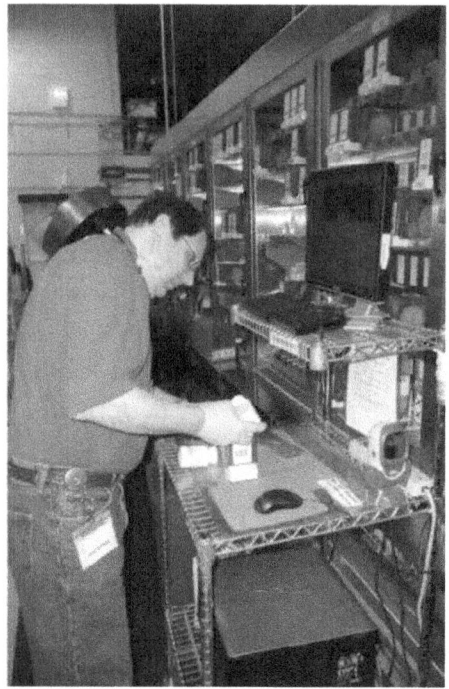

Figure 4. Employee replenishing an Optifill canister with the Optifill machine in the background.

of the eight shared chutes in each machine. A canister dispensed the appropriate pharmaceutical into the chute that funneled into the bottle. The Optifill machine filled approximately 2,000 prescriptions per day during our evaluation. Two pharmacy technicians replenished and repaired the Optifill canisters. A pharmacist checked and verified all replenishments.

Some employees also worked in the repack, special handling, or manual count areas in the warehouse. Pharmacy technicians in the repack area filled multiple prescriptions of the same pharmaceutical using another automatic dispensing machine. One pharmacy technician transferred pharmaceuticals from bottles into larger totes. The contents of the totes were dumped into the hopper of the repack machine. The machine used vibration plates to feed the bottles. Use of the repack machine was permanently discontinued shortly after our first visit. A pharmacy technician in the special handling area primarily filled prescriptions of warfarin by hand. In the manual count area, two or three pharmacy technicians hand filled a variety of other prescriptions. On rare occasions, these pharmacy technicians filled prescriptions of hazardous drugs. Hazardous drugs are drugs known or suspected to cause adverse health effects from exposures in the workplace [NIOSH 2004, 2010a]. The hand filling of hazardous drugs was moved to a separate area with dedicated personnel shortly before our second visit.

During a night shift on our first visit, we observed the cleaning of the Optifill and Baker machines by four pharmacy technicians. The Optifill machine was cleaned by opening the cabinet doors, collecting pharmaceutical dust on the chutes with a HEPA vacuum, and then wiping the chutes with alcohol. The Baker machine was cleaned by emptying pharmaceuticals contained in a cell into a tote, disassembling and repairing any broken cell parts, and then cleaning the inside of the cell with alcohol and a dry wipe before reassembly. The pharmaceuticals held in the tote were then dumped back into the clean cell.

The purpose of this evaluation was to (1) determine if and during which activities dust was released into the air, (2) measure the concentration of the airborne dust, (3) determine if the airborne dust contained pharmaceuticals, (4) identify and quantify specific APIs in the airborne dust, (5) determine if employees were experiencing or at risk of adverse health effects related to their exposures, (6) measure production employees' full-shift personal noise exposures to determine if hearing protection was needed, and (7) measure sound levels and noise frequency levels near equipment to help identify possible noise control approaches. Bilingual NIOSH investigators fluent in Spanish aided our communication with Hispanic employees during this evaluation.

Air Sampling

The methods we used to measure PBZ concentrations of total, respirable, and inhalable dust are summarized in Table 1. During the second visit, the total dust and inhalable dust samplers were positioned side by side in the employees' PBZs. Each type of dust sampler collects particles in different size ranges. A respirable dust sampler has 50% collection efficiency for particles with an aerodynamic diameter of 4 μm. These respirable particles are able to penetrate deeply into the lower respiratory system [ACGIH 2011]. An inhalable dust sampler collects larger particles than a total dust sampler (with closed-face configuration) because it has a larger inlet. An inhalable dust sampler has 50% collection efficiency for particles with an aerodynamic diameter of 100 μm. These inhalable particles can be deposited anywhere in the respiratory system, including the nose [ACGIH 2011].

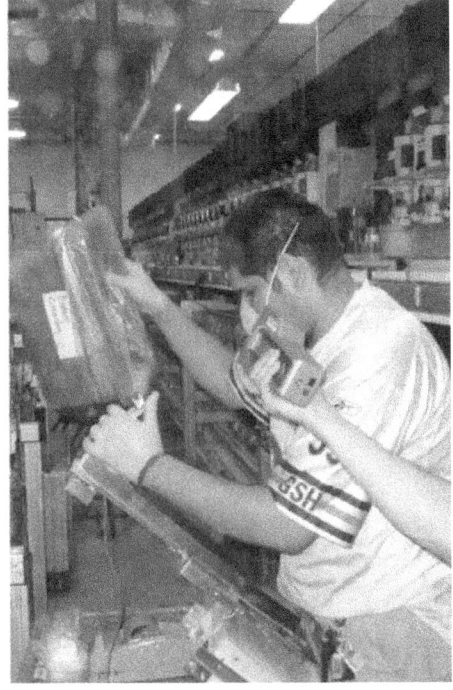

Figure 5. Using a real-time particle meter to measure particle counts near the PBZ of an employee cleaning a Baker cell.

Real-time particle count measurements were collected near the PBZs of the employees during different tasks (Figure 5). These measurements along with the real-time PBZ concentrations of respirable dust were used to identify specific tasks that resulted in increased particle counts. The types of tablets that were handled during the releases of dust were recorded. Managers and employees at the pharmacy also provided us with a list of tablets that were especially dusty. Generally, capsules did not produce dust. Using this information, we generated lists of APIs that could potentially be present on each total dust air filter. More information about the dust sampling methods and particle count measurements is provided in Appendix A.

Table 1. Summary of the initial air sampling and analyses performed at the mail order pharmacy

Sampling media/equipment*	Flow rate (Lpm)	Analytes	NIOSH analytical method[†]	Personal air sampling	
				N[‡]	n[§]
First visit					
37-mm PTFE filter, closed face cassette	4	Total dust (by mass)	0500	22	35
37-mm PTFE filter, cyclone, Personal DataRAM	2.2	Respirable dust (by mass and in real time)	0600	4	6
HHPC-6 optical particle counter	NA	Particle count (in real time)	NA	NA	NA
Second visit					
37-mm PTFE filter, closed face cassette	4	Total dust (by mass)	0500	11	25
25-mm PTFE filter, IOM sampler	2	Inhalable dust (by mass)	0600	11	25
HHPC-6 optical particle counter	NA	Particle count (in real time)	NA	NA	NA

* Additional information provided in Appendix A.
[†] NIOSH Manual of Analytical Methods [NIOSH 2011]
[‡] Number of employees sampled
[§] Total number of air samples

Figure 6 illustrates the progression of other analyses done on the total and inhalable dust filters after they were analyzed gravimetrically. The NIOSH contract laboratory, BVNA (Novi, Michigan), quantified lactose, a common excipient (nonactive ingredient) in pharmaceuticals, on the inhalable dust filters using an internal analytical method. The total dust air filters were sent to Prosolia, Inc. (Indianapolis, Indiana) along with the lists of APIs likely to be present on each filter. Prosolia used a DESI/MS system [Takats et al. 2004] to identify specific APIs on the filters by cross referencing mass-to-charge ratios with the lists of APIs we provided.

We used the list of identified APIs and real-time air sampling results to select inhalable dust samples (collected side by side with the total dust air samples) for further analysis. We selected five inhalable dust samples for quantitation of lisinopril. Lisinopril was chosen for quantitation because the analytical method used by BVNA requires dissolution in water, and the inhalable dust samples were already dissolved in water for the lactose analysis. In addition, lisinopril has a relatively low manufacturer's OEL of 10 $\mu g/m^3$ [Bristol-Myers Squibb Company 2008]. We also selected five total dust air samples for quantitation of warfarin using NIOSH Method 5002 [NIOSH 2011]. We chose to analyze for warfarin because it was the predominant drug handled by the employees in the manual count (special handling) area. The analytical methods used to quantify lactose and lisinopril are summarized in Appendix A.

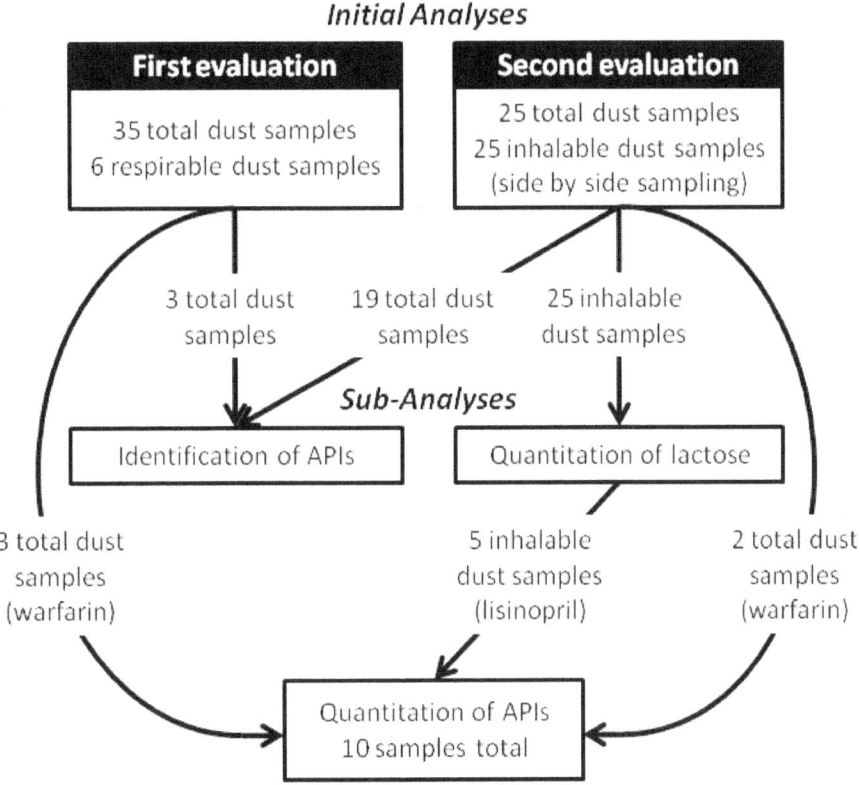

Figure 6. Flow chart showing the subanalyses performed on the total and inhalable dust samples.

Medical Interviews

During our first visit, we conducted voluntary confidential medical interviews with a convenience sample of employees. The interviews focused on respiratory and skin symptoms as well as perceived exposure to dust and noise. We spoke to all 23 Baker and Optifill operators and to a comparable number of employees from other locations.

Noise Measurements

During the second visit, we collected 36 full-shift TWA personal noise dosimetry measurements and 3 full-shift TWA area noise dosimetry measurements. We measured area noise levels and performed octave band noise frequency analysis (measurement of noise levels in different frequencies) at noisy equipment and work areas with a Larson Davis (Depew, New York) System 824 sound level meter and real-time frequency analyzer. Appendix A provides more information on the noise measurements.

RESULTS

Exposure to Pharmaceutical Dust

Figures 7 and 8 summarize the PBZ total dust (ranging from 31–530 $\mu g/m^3$) and respirable dust (ranging from ND–33 $\mu g/m^3$) concentrations from the first visit. Figure 9 summarizes the PBZ inhalable dust (ranging from 110–800 $\mu g/m^3$), total dust (ranging from 6–260 $\mu g/m^3$), and lactose concentrations (ranging from 0.94–63 $\mu g/m^3$) from the second visit. Exposures to employees who maintained the Baker machine were stratified by the tasks they performed most (cleaning Baker cells versus maintaining the machine). This was done because exposure levels varied substantially between those two tasks. General area air concentrations (measured in the non-production areas of the pharmacy) are also included in Figure 9 to show the relatively low background levels of dust and lactose. Standard deviations are represented by error bars in all the figures. The MDCs and MQCs were calculated by dividing the analytical limits of detection and quantitation (mass units) by the average volume of air sampled. The MDCs and MQCs represent the smallest air concentrations that could have been detected (MDC) or quantified (MQC) on the basis of the volume of air sampled. Non-detectable levels of respirable dust were imputed values calculated by dividing their MDC of 20 $\mu g/m^3$ by the square root of 2 [Hornung and Reed 1990].

The total dust concentrations were similar between the two visits. However, the total dust concentration measured during the cleaning of Baker cells during the first visit was higher than that measured on the second visit. During the first visit, we collected total and respirable dust samples on employees doing similar processes, and the average total dust concentrations were 4 times higher than the respirable dust concentrations. During the second visit, the average inhalable dust concentrations were 1.3 to 3.7 times higher than the average total dust concentrations measured on the same employees. Lactose was a small fraction (0.08%–13%) of the inhalable dust, but was quantified in all inhalable dust air samples. Area air concentrations of lactose in the non-production areas of the pharmacy were significantly lower ($P < 0.001$) than the PBZ concentrations measured on employees in the production areas.

Other than the night shift, the total dust exposures overall were greater for employees in the warehouse than in the pharmacy during both visits. Inhalable dust exposures measured during the second visit were similar between the warehouse and pharmacy employees. During the second visit, the highest average total and inhalable dust exposures were measured in the PBZs of employees who did offline replenishment of Baker canisters, hand filling of prescriptions (manual count), online replenishment of Optifill canisters, and cleaning of Baker cells. Employees doing these processes, as well as the hand filling of prescriptions (special handling), also had the highest average PBZ concentrations of lactose.

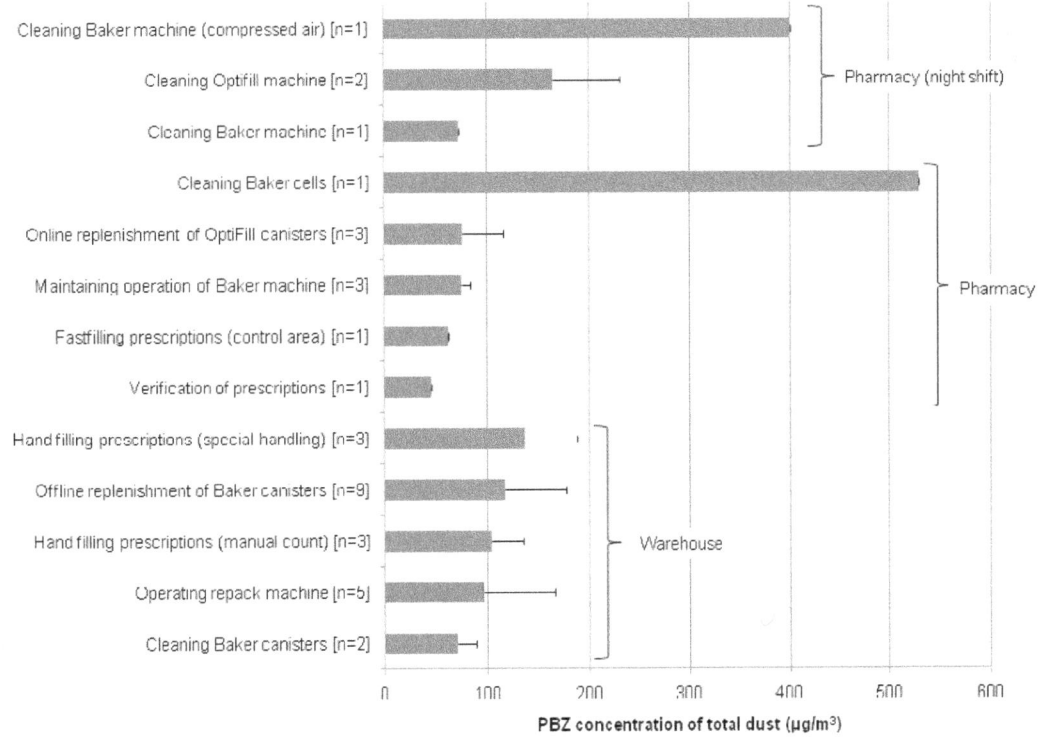

Figure 7. Summary of average work-shift (approximately 8 hours) PBZ concentrations of total dust measured during the first visit by process and location at the facility. (Note: The night shift samples were task-based samples collected over 80 to 130 minutes.)

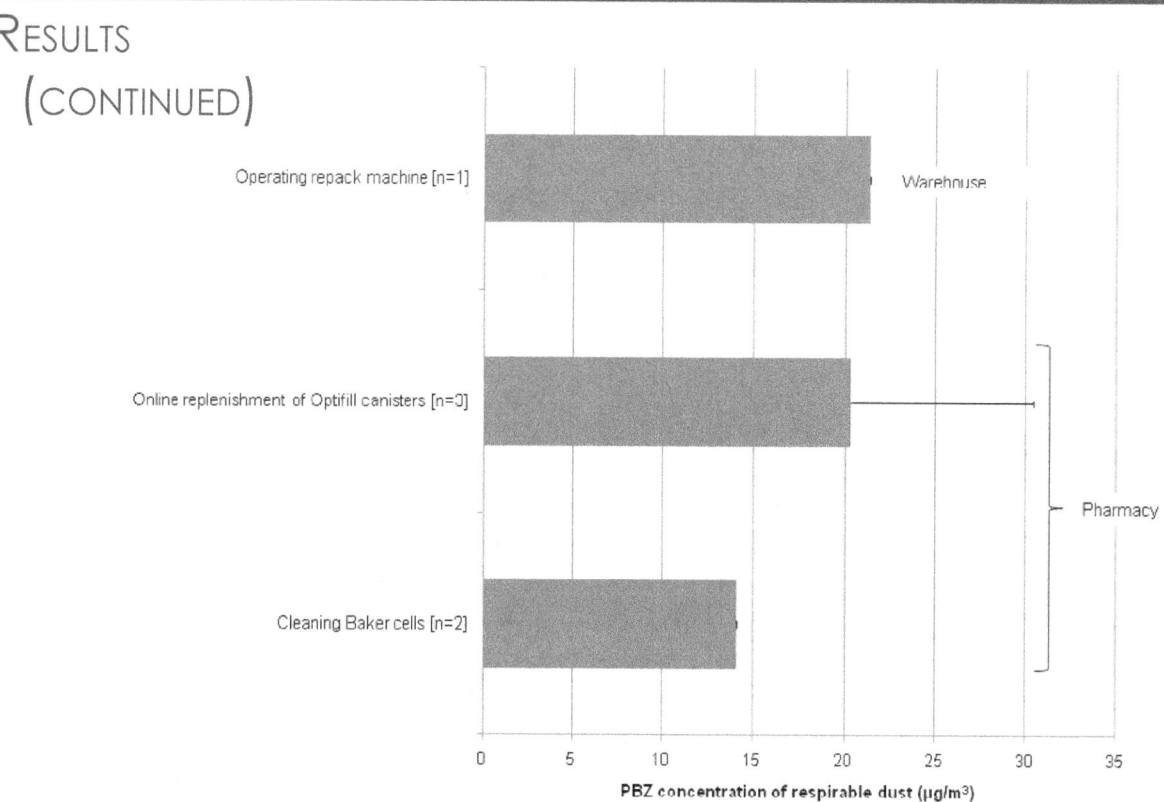

Figure 8. Summary of average work-shift PBZ concentrations of respirable dust measured during the first visit by process and location at the facility.

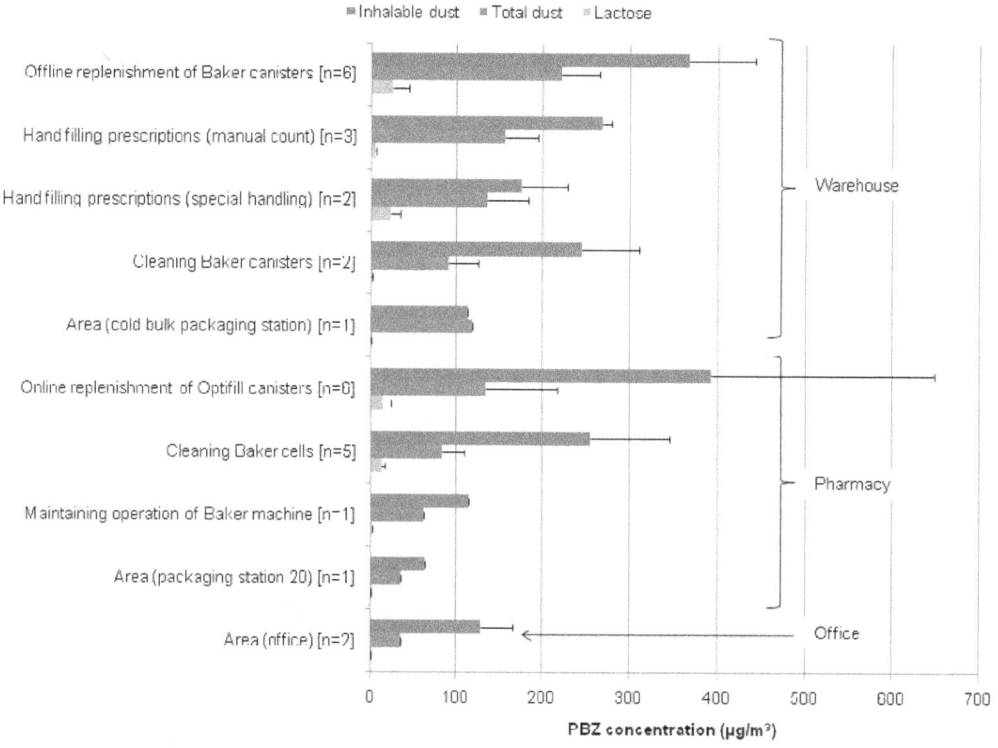

Figure 9. Summary of average work-shift PBZ concentrations of inhalable dust, total dust, and lactose measured during the second visit by process and location at the facility.

Results
(continued)

Figures 10 and 11 show the real-time respirable particle concentrations, and Figures 12–15 show the real-time particle counts measured over time in the PBZs of employees doing different processes. The work-shift or task-based PBZ dust concentrations are also provided in these figures. Peaks in particle concentrations and counts were correlated with different tasks involving specific APIs. These APIs are noted in the figures above the corresponding peaks. Only tasks involving tablets were correlated with releases of dust. Because the respirable dust concentrations were so low (ND–33 µg/m³), only the total dust samples were sent for further analysis for specific APIs. The names of the APIs in Figures 12–15 that were identified using DESI/MS on the corresponding PBZ total dust samples are shown in red ovals. Although submicron (0.3–1 µm) particles dominated the particle counts (Figures 12–15), these small particles have negligible mass. Thus, the larger particles (>3 µm) contributed substantially more mass on the total and inhalable dust air samples than the small particles.

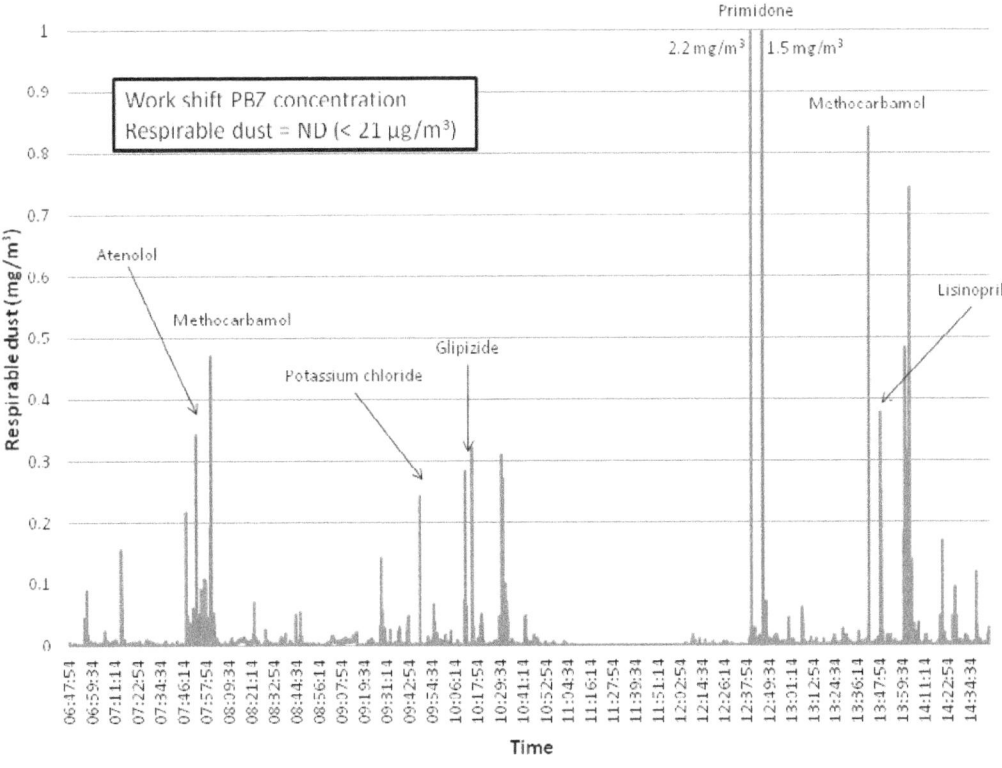

Figure 10. Real-time respirable dust concentrations measured in the PBZ of Employee 7 who cleaned Baker cells as needed throughout the work day (April 6, 2010). The APIs contained in the cells that Employee 7 cleaned are noted above the peaks in respirable dust concentrations that occurred at the same time.

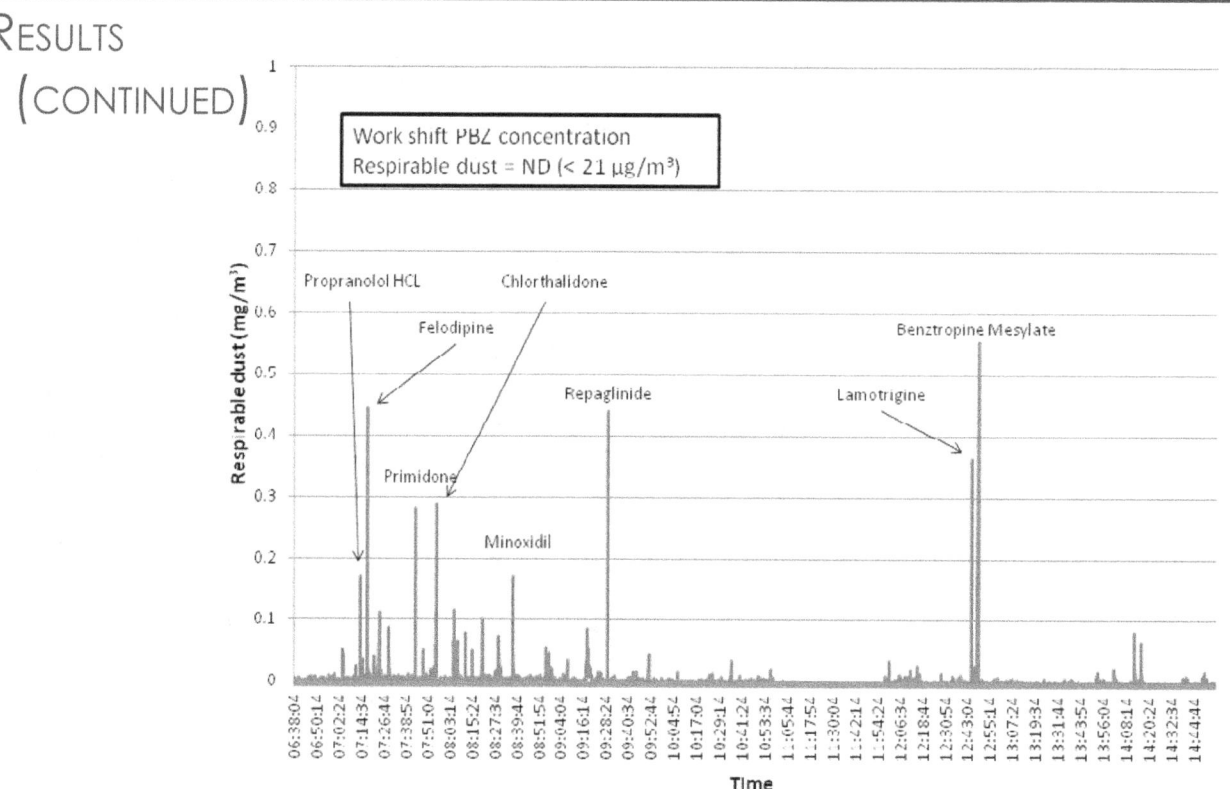

Figure 11. Real-time respirable dust concentrations measured in the PBZ of Employee 6 who performed online replenishment of Optifill canisters throughout the work day (April 7, 2010). The APIs that Employee 6 handled during replenishment of the cells are noted above the peaks in respirable dust concentrations that occurred at the same time.

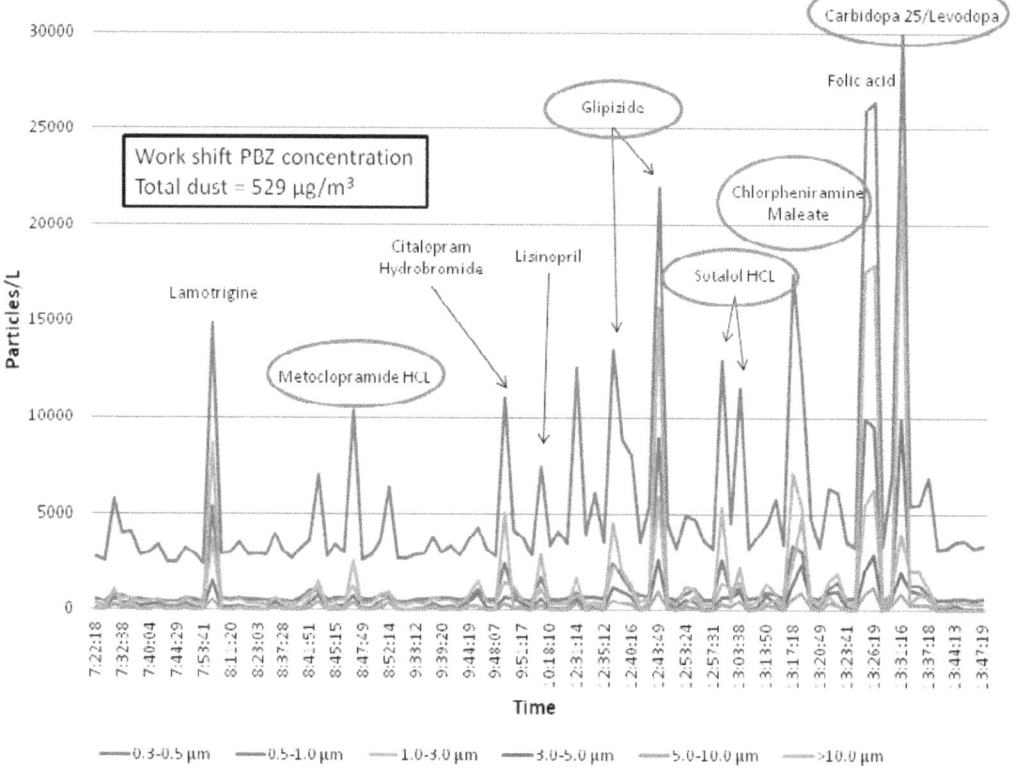

Figure 12. Real-time particle counts measured near the PBZ of Employee 7 who cleaned Baker cells as needed throughout the work day (April 8, 2010). The APIs contained in the cells that Employee 7 cleaned are noted above the peaks in particle counts that occurred at the same time. The names of the APIs identified on the corresponding total dust air sample are shown in the red ovals.

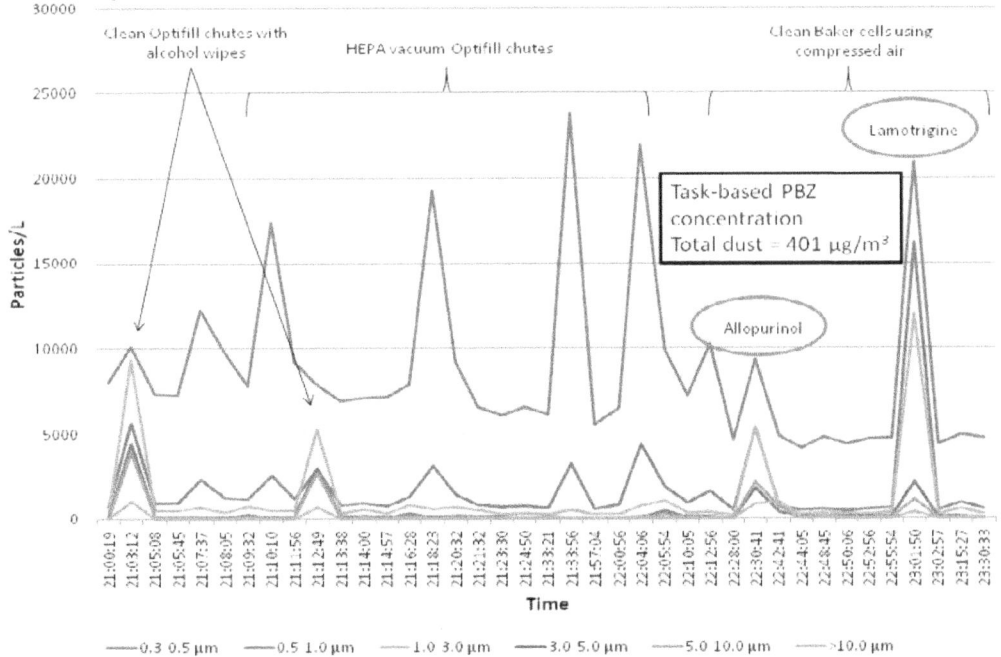

Figure 13. Real-time particle counts measured near the PBZs of employees who cleaned the Optifill machine (Employees 4 and 25) and the Baker machine (Employee 10) during the night shift on April 7, 2010. The task-based PBZ concentration of total dust is provided for Employee 10. The APIs contained in the cells that Employee 10 cleaned with compressed air are noted above the peaks in particle counts that occurred at the same time. The names of the APIs identified on the corresponding total dust air sample are shown in the red ovals.

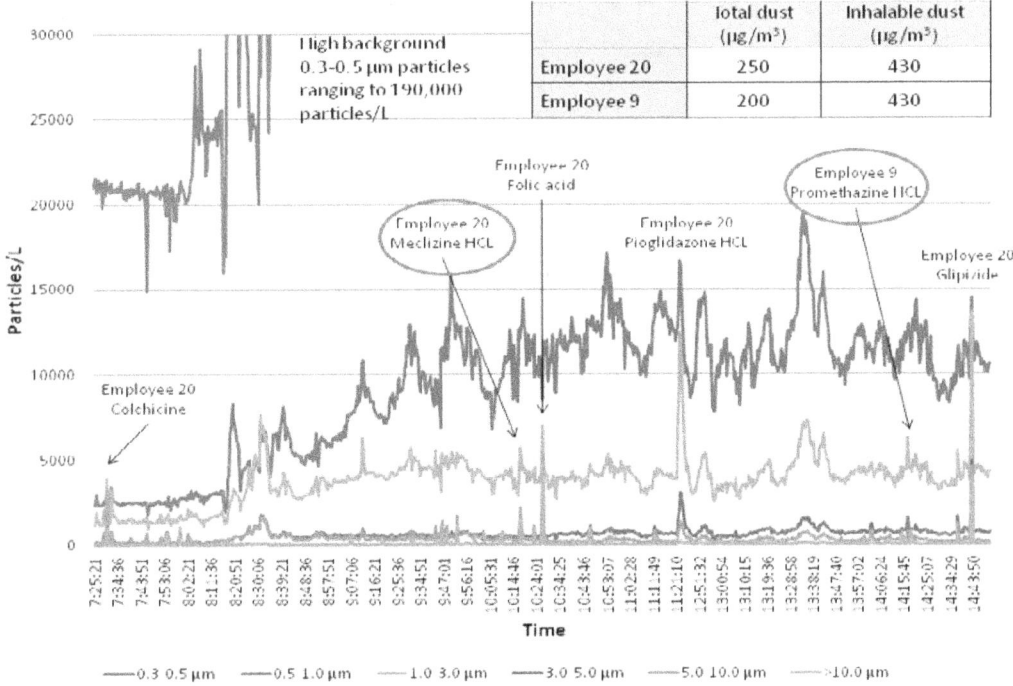

Figure 14. Real-time particle counts measured near the PBZs of Employees 9 and 20 (who worked near each other) during the offline replenishment of Baker canisters on December 7, 2010. The APIs that were handled during the filling of the canisters (and employees who handled them) are noted above the peaks in particle counts that occurred at the same time. The names of the APIs identified on the corresponding total dust air samples are shown in the red ovals.

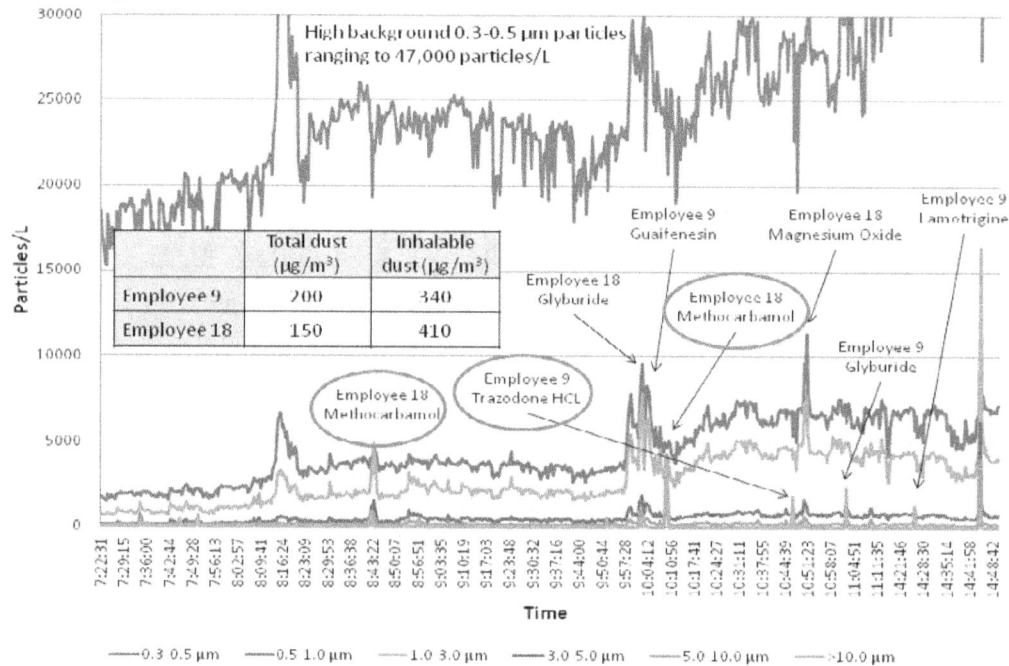

Figure 15. Real-time particle counts measured near the PBZs of Employees 9 and 18 during the offline replenishment of Baker canisters on December 8, 2010. The APIs that were handled during the filling of the canisters (and the employees who handled them) are noted above the peaks in particle counts that occurred at the same time. The names of the APIs identified on the corresponding total dust air samples are shown in the red ovals.

The 22 APIs identified on the total dust filters using DESI/MS are shown in Table 2. Appendix B provides more information on these APIs, their therapeutic uses, and manufacturers' OELs (if available). Table 3 contains the PBZ air concentrations for warfarin and lisinopril. The PBZ concentrations of warfarin, measured during the hand filling of warfarin prescriptions (special handling), ranged from 0.19–3.8 $\mu g/m^3$ and were well below the NIOSH REL, OSHA PEL, and ACGIH TLV of 100 $\mu g/m^3$ [ACGIH 2001, NIOSH 2010b]. Likewise, the PBZ concentrations of lisinopril, measured during different processes, ranged from ND–0.44 $\mu g/m^3$ and were well below the manufacturer's OEL of 10 $\mu g/m^3$ [Bristol-Myers Squibb Company 2008].

Use of Surgical Masks, Respirators, and Protective Clothing

During our first visit, we observed several employees voluntarily wearing employer-provided surgical masks and dust masks (Medline Prohibit NON27381, Figure 4) that were not NIOSH-approved respirators. Employees believed that these masks protected them from exposure to the pharmaceutical dust. Surgical

Table 2. APIs identified on the total dust air samples using DESI/MS analysis (X denotes that the compound was identified in that sample)

Process	Employee ID	Date	Allopurinol	Benazepril	Bethanechol	Buspirone	Carbidopa	Chlorpheniramine	Doxazosin	Glipizide	Hydralazine	Lamotrigine	Levodopa	Lisinopril	Meclizine	Metformin	Methocarbamol	Metoclopramide	Naproxen	Oxybutynin	Promethazine	Sotalol	Trazadone	Venlafaxine
Operating repack machine	3	4/8/2010																	X					X
Checking online replenishment of Optifill canisters	6	12/7/2010										X			X									
		12/8/2010																						
		12/9/2010		X								X			X									
Cleaning Baker cells	7	4/8/2010					X	X		X								X				X		
		12/7/2010																				X		
		12/8/2010																				X	X	
		12/9/2010				X					X					X								
Offline replenishment of Baker canisters	9	12/7/2010																			X			
		12/8/2010														X	X						X	
Cleaning Baker machine (night shift)	10	4/7/2010	X								X													
Online replenishment of Optifill canisters	16	12/7/2010							X			X			X									X
		12/8/2010										X			X									X
		12/9/2010													X									
Hand filling of prescriptions (manual count)	17	12/7/2010																						X
		12/9/2010																						
Offline replenishment of Baker canisters	18	12/8/2010															X						X	
Offline replenishment of Baker canisters	20	12/7/2010													X									
		12/9/2010								X														
Cleaning Baker cells	21	12/7/2010										X	X	X										
		12/8/2010			X											X				X				
Offline replenishment of Baker canisters	24	12/9/2010								X													X	

Table 3. Personal breathing zone air concentrations of warfarin and lisinopril for employees who handled these tablets

Process	Employee ID	Date	Warfarin (µg/m³) (total dust)	Lisinopril (µg/m³) (inhalable dust)
Hand filling prescriptions (special handling)	8	4/8/2010	3.8	
	11	4/6/2010	(0.19)	
	11	4/7/2010	3.1	
	23	12/8/2010	(0.64)	
	23	12/9/2010	(0.50)	
Cleaning Baker cells	7	12/7/2010		(0.44)
	7	12/8/2010		ND
	7	12/9/2010		ND
	21	12/7/2010		ND
Offline replenishment of Baker canisters	9	12/7/2010		ND
OEL			100*	10†
MDC			0.18–0.42	0.22
MQC			0.59–2.2	0.69

* NIOSH REL, OSHA PEL, and ACGIH TLV [NIOSH 2010b, ACGIH 2011]
† Manufacturer's OEL [Bristol-Myers Squibb Company 2008]

masks are designed to protect nearby people, or as in this case, pharmaceuticals, from expectorated droplets released by the person wearing the mask. Some employees were wearing the dust masks incorrectly (upside down). We informed the employer about these observations and noted that the employer could allow voluntary use of respirators for employee protection but would need to follow the requirements in the OSHA respiratory protection standard [29 CFR 1910.134] pertaining to voluntary respirator use, such as providing employees with the standard's Appendix D, "Information for Employees Using Respirators When Not Required Under the Standard." We also recommended that they provide three sizes of at least two different models of NIOSH approved N95 filtering facepiece respirators and provide training on how to properly wear and maintain these respirators.

By our second visit, the pharmacy had implemented some of these recommendations. Employees were provided with Appendix D of the OSHA respiratory protection standard [29 CFR 1910.134]. Two different models of N95 filtering facepiece respirators (Moldex

220N95 and Moldex 2300N95) were available to employees. At least two different respirator sizes were available, but many employees did not know where to access them. Instead employees typically used the model and size respirator in their work area. Only sick employees were required to wear surgical masks to protect the pharmaceuticals from contamination. We still observed that some employees wore the respirators incorrectly. In particular, a few employees wore a respirator that was either too small or large for their facial structure and thus did not seal against their faces, limiting the protection afforded by the respirator. In addition, some employees were not properly storing their respirators. We recommend putting respirators in a bag or container between uses to prevent contamination of the interior of the respirator.

Most employees wore either vinyl examination gloves (0.14–0.17 mm thickness) or nitrile gloves (0.12–0.18 mm thickness) when handling pharmaceuticals. The employees who did offline replenishment of the Baker cells also wore hair nets. In addition, a few employees who hand filled prescriptions wore cloth aprons.

Dispensing of Hazardous Drugs

The pharmacy stocked 61 hazardous drugs as per the NIOSH list of hazardous drugs [NIOSH 2010a], 35 of which were tablets and therefore potentially capable of producing dust. Of all the hazardous drugs, estrogen was probably distributed in the highest volumes with the Optifill machine. This estrogen medication was a low dose (< 0.625 mg) tablet; we did not identify it in any of the total dust air samples collected from the employees who replenished the Optifill canisters. The other hazardous drugs were distributed infrequently in the manual count area of the warehouse during our first visit. The manual count employees were instructed by the employer to wear nitrile gloves and N95 filtering facepiece respirators when filling hazardous drug prescriptions. This was the same policy for the special handling employees who primarily worked with warfarin. By our second visit, the N95 filtering facepiece respirators were no longer mandated in these areas, but were being used as part of a voluntary use program. The pharmacy did not have written standard operating procedures for work involving hazardous drugs until our second visit. These procedures required hazardous drug prescriptions to be filled and verified in a separate area by employees wearing gloves and gave directions on what to do in case a drug was spilled. No other control measures were required.

Other Observations

During the first visit, we observed the use of compressed air to clean Baker cells during the night shift, which resulted in the second highest PBZ total dust concentration. Pharmacy managers told us that this activity was prohibited, and we did not observe this activity during the day shift. We also observed white dust on surfaces at work stations (Figure 16) that may have been from pharmaceuticals. We noticed that many employees washed hands before eating; however, we did not carefully observe hand washing during our evaluation. Most, if not all, employees wore their work outfits when they left the worksite.

Health Symptoms

We interviewed 45 employees (31 first shift and 14 second shift employees). Seventeen worked on or near the Baker machine, and six worked on or near the Optifill machine. Twenty-four were female, with a mean age of 36 years. Eleven were pharmacy employees, and 34 were contractors. The job titles were as follows: 9 shipping-packers, 28 pharmacy technicians, 4 pharmacists, and 1 each housekeeper, material handler, cell maintenance technician, and labeler. Their mean employment duration was 5 years. Of the 23 Optifill and Baker machine employees, 19 said they were exposed to dust, 12 specifically to dust from drugs. Sixteen of the other employees said they were exposed to dust, seven specifically to dust from drugs. Twenty-one employees, seven of whom worked on or near the Baker or Optifill machines, reported eye and upper respiratory irritation. Noise was a concern in certain areas, such as near the Optifill bottle hoppers and at the end of the packing line. Heat in the summer was a common concern, especially in the warehouse area.

Exposures to Noise

One pharmacy technician working at the Baker machine had a TWA noise exposure that was above the OSHA AL and NIOSH REL of 85 dBA (Table 4). All other monitored employees' TWA noise exposures were less than OSHA and NIOSH exposure limits. TWA noise exposures at the ADU labeling machine, offline replenishment, packing station and verification area were less than 80 dBA.

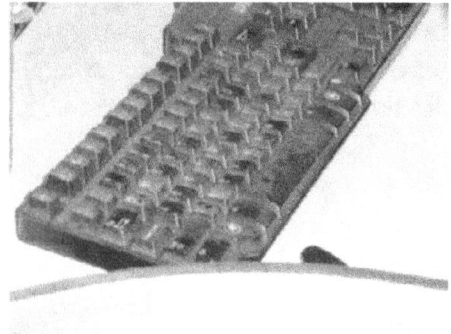

Figure 16. White dust covering a computer keyboard at the workstation of an employee who did offline replenishment of Baker cells.

RESULTS (CONTINUED)

One-third octave band noise level measurements from several work areas or pieces of equipment are shown Figure 17. The predominant noise frequencies for most were greater than 8,000 Hz. In contrast, the highest noise levels at pharmacy station #5 were at 630 Hz and 25 Hz. In addition to high noise levels above 8,000 Hz, the capper also had a noise level peak at 125 Hz. The Optifill had a secondary peak at 630–800 Hz, and the other work areas had secondary peaks at frequencies below 500 Hz.

Table 4. Summary of TWA noise exposure measurements

Work area or equipment	Job title	N	NIOSH REL (dBA)	OSHA AL (dBA)	OSHA PEL (dBA)
ADU labeling machine	Technician	2	75.5 – 77.8	67.9 – 72.1	56.2 – 59.0
Baker	Technician	10	81.1 – 88.2	77.7 – 85.1	63.9 – 80.2
	Pharmacist	4	77.4 – 80.6	73.2 – 75.8	49.3 – 60.9
	Area sample	1	79.0	76.1	32.4
Labeling	Team leader	2	79.9 – 81.6	76.1 – 78.1	60.5 – 65.3
	Technician	5	69.9 – 81.2	58.0 – 77.7	46.9 – 65.1
Offline replenishment	Technician	1	70.1	55.7	52.1
	Area sample	2	65.5 – 65.9	50.3 – 51.1	41.6 – 41.8
Optifill	Pharmacist	2	77.0 – 80.7	73.1 – 74.8	47.1 – 68.0
Packing station	Packer	6	69.4 – 78.5	57.8 – 73.7	39.6 – 60.1
Verification	Pharmacist	3	71.8 – 77.5	64.9 – 72.4	36.8 – 58.0
Noise Exposure Limits			85	85	90

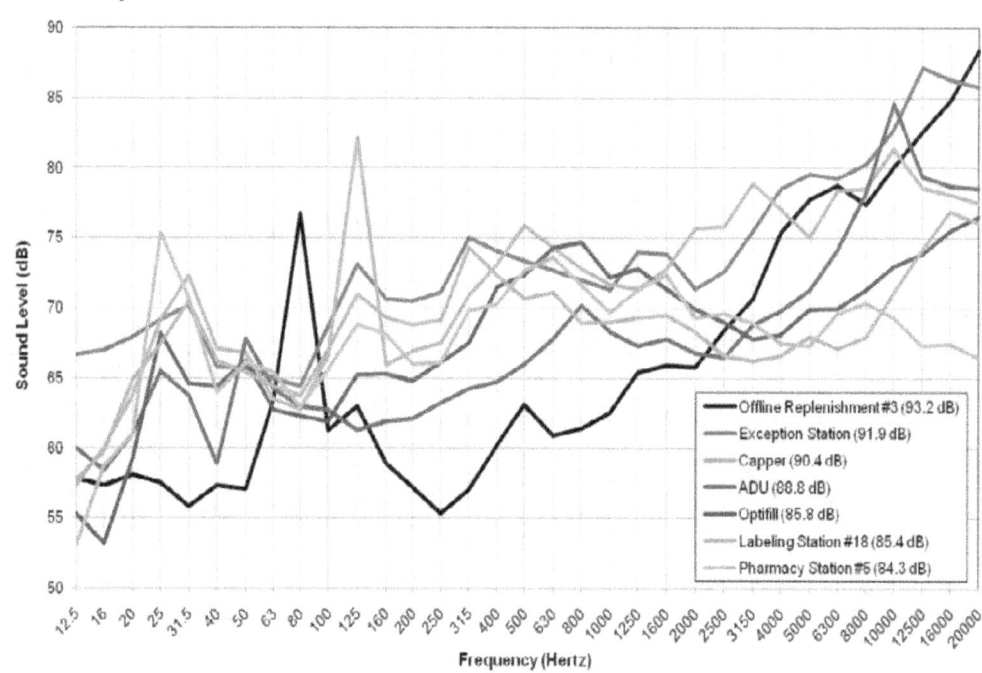

Figure 17: Octave band noise frequency measurement results (unweighted sound levels shown in parentheses).

DISCUSSION

Several tasks involving the handling of tablets correlated with peaks in real-time respirable particle concentration (Figures 10 and 11) and particle counts (Figures 12–15), suggesting that pharmaceutical dust was released into the air where it could be inhaled by employees. The low levels of respirable dust suggest that respirable particles did not contribute substantially to the dust concentrations. Total dust samplers (with closed-face configuration) have been shown to under sample particles larger than 30 μm in aerodynamic diameter [Kenny et al. 1997]. Thus, the higher levels of inhalable dust compared to total dust that we found suggest that some particles >30 μm were released. When inhaled, these larger particles are likely to be captured in the upper respiratory tract [Hinds 1999]. These larger particles also settle quickly to the ground. Thus, much of the pharmaceutical dust that was released probably did not stay suspended in the air for more than a few seconds.

Occupational exposure limits for general dust or particles not otherwise regulated are only applicable when the dust particles are biologically inert and are insoluble in water [ACGIH 2011].

DISCUSSION (CONTINUED)

Pharmaceutical dust does not meet these criteria because APIs are designed to elicit biological responses, and most tablets are water soluble. Our data suggest that at least some of the dust we collected on air samples came from pharmaceuticals. Lactose, a common excipient in pharmaceuticals, was present in all inhalable dust air samples, and specific APIs were identified in most of the total dust air samples. Moreover, we selected two APIs (warfarin and lisinopril) for quantitation in air and found them to be present in one or more air samples. The solubility of pharmaceuticals in water could cause inhaled particles to be systemically absorbed in the upper respiratory tract. If not absorbed, some of the particles would be cleared to the esophagus and ingested [Hinds 1999]. Therefore, it is not appropriate to compare the PBZ dust concentrations we measured to the OELs for particles not otherwise specified or regulated.

The PBZ air concentrations of warfarin and lisinopril did not exceed their respective OELs. The NIOSH REL, OSHA PEL, and ACGIH TLV for warfarin are intended to minimize the potential for hemorrhage of biological tissues, such as mucous membranes [ACGIH 2001, NIOSH 2010b]. The manufacturer's OEL for lisinopril [Bristol-Myers Squibb Company 2008] was established using a control banding process that considers a variety of toxicological data. See Appendix B for more information about control banding in the pharmaceutical industry.

Allergic reactions and upper respiratory irritation are probably the most likely health effects from inhalation exposure to low levels of APIs (well below therapeutic doses). Most of the employees interviewed did not report having work-related health effects. When symptoms were reported, they were compatible with general exposure to dust (i.e., eye and upper-respiratory irritation). Exposure to APIs could also contribute to these symptoms.

We believe it is prudent to reduce exposures to pharmaceutical dust for the following reasons:

1. Employees are being exposed to low levels of APIs that they were not prescribed. Moreover, they are inhaling these APIs rather than ingesting them, which could change how the chemical affects the body.

2. Some individuals may be allergic to specific APIs or may be taking medications that could interact with APIs that they inhale at work.

3. We cannot be certain that exposures to all the APIs did not exceed OELs or acceptable levels. We quantified only two of the 22 APIs that we identified in air. In addition, not all APIs have published OELs. The absence of an OEL does not mean the chemical is safe.

4. The potential health effects from exposures to multiple APIs are unknown. We identified as many as five APIs on one total dust air sample. It is possible that one API could enhance the effect of another API, although allergic reactions and upper respiratory irritation are the most likely health effects.

5. Pharmaceutical dust is likely to contaminate surfaces (Figure 16) and clothing. If employees do not wear gloves or wash hands before eating or using tobacco products as mandated, they could ingest APIs. Dermal absorption is also possible depending on the chemical makeup of APIs. Secondary exposure to family members could occur if personal clothing becomes contaminated with pharmaceutical dust and is worn at home. Children may be especially susceptible to adverse health effects from API exposures [Brent et al. 2004].

At this mail order pharmacy, exposure to hazardous drugs (per the NIOSH list of hazardous drugs [NIOSH 2010a]) presents the greatest potential health risk to pharmacy employees. Most of these drugs were dispensed manually, although at least one hormone medication (estrogen) was dispensed in the Optifill machine. Without proper precautions, exposures can occur when hazardous drugs are handled, particularly if these drugs are in tablet form and capable of producing dust. Exposures to hazardous drugs, even at low levels, can lead to serious health effects including skin rashes, reproductive problems, and possibly cancer [NIOSH 2004]. To provide employees with the greatest protection, employers should implement necessary engineering and administrative controls and ensure that employees use sound procedures for handling hazardous drugs and proper protective equipment [NIOSH 2004].

While most of the hazardous drugs were handled in a designated area, the other pharmaceuticals of varying toxicity were handled throughout the mail order pharmacy. Therefore, prioritization of control measures for work involving these pharmaceuticals should be based on the dust levels observed during different processes. In general, employees who cleaned cells, replenished canisters, and hand filled prescriptions had the highest PBZ concentrations of

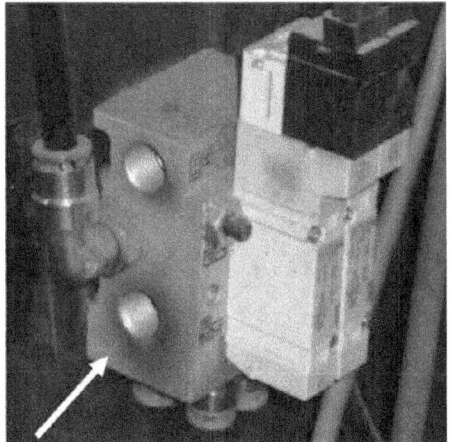

Figure 18. Exhaust ports of a solenoid valve without silencing mufflers.

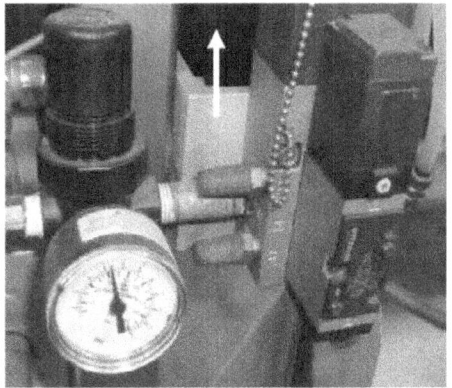

Figure 19. Mufflers on an exhaust port of a solenoid valve.

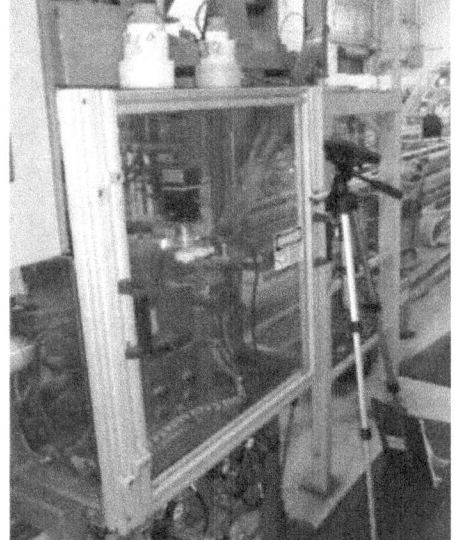

Figure 20. The capper unit enclosure.

total dust, inhalable dust, and lactose. The potential for exposure to pharmaceutical dust also existed during the operation of the repack machine, particularly when tablets were dumped into totes and when the totes were emptied into the machine, but the use of the repack machine was discontinued shortly after our first visit.

For some work areas, such as the offline replenishment, exception station, and Baker machine, high frequency noise was generated by compressed air exhausting from solenoid valves and actuators. For most of the solenoid valves, compressed air was exhausted directly out of the exhaust port (Figure 18), generating substantial high frequency noise from air turbulence as the compressed air exited the exhaust port. However, a few of the exhaust ports had mufflers (Figure 19) to reduce noise. Additionally, reducing the pressure in the compressed air system may help reduce noise levels. In a few work areas, such as the offline replenishment, leaking compressed air also generated noise. Identification and repair of leaks in the compressed air system will eliminate this noise.

The capper, located near the west side of the Baker machine, generated a high frequency noise when caps were screwed onto prescription bottles and was a major source of noise in that area. The capper had an enclosure around most of the unit (Figure 20). Equipment enclosures are a common and often useful approach for controlling and reducing high frequency noise exposures. However, the capper was not enclosed on the bottom and had thin gaps along the corners and a small opening in the side panel (Figure 21) for prescription bottles to pass through. Adding a bottom panel, sealing the gaps along the corners, and reducing the size of any opening may reduce noise levels near the capper.

Noise at the Optifill bottler was generated by a short burst of compressed air released when a bottle was not properly aligned. In addition, the burst of air propelled the bottle and caused it to strike the hard plastic cover of the Optifill machine. Reduction of air pressure may reduce noise from the compressed air burst and prevent prescription bottles from striking the cover. Additionally, using a thicker plastic cover on the Optifill machine will dampen the sound if a bottle does hit the cover.

Some work areas, particularly the capper, offline replenishment, and pharmacy station, had high noise levels in low frequencies (< 500 Hz). Low frequency noise is commonly caused by equipment vibration. Unlike high frequency noise, machine enclosures are

DISCUSSION (CONTINUED)

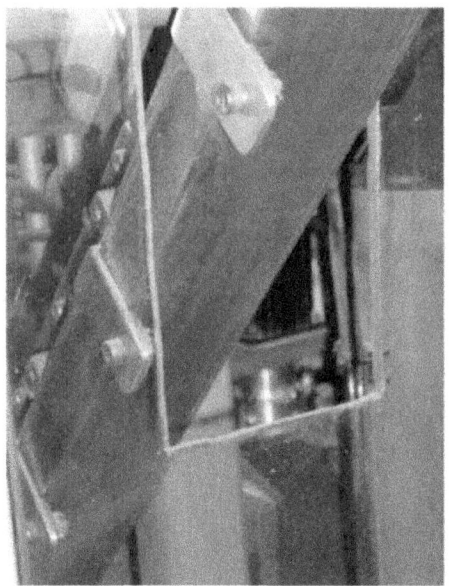

Figure 21. Opening in the side panel of the capper enclosure.

not effective in reducing low frequency noise. Noise reduction strategies for low frequency noise should focus on reducing equipment vibration. For example, installing appropriately designed vibration isolation pads or springs can reduce vibration transmitted from operating equipment to surrounding surfaces.

A few employees wore foam insert hearing protection, but most of those wearing hearing protection did not insert the hearing protectors deeply enough into their ear canal. The hearing protectors provided by the employer had a noise reduction rating of 29 dB, which is more noise reduction than is actually needed for the noise levels in the facility. When hearing protectors reduce noise more than necessary, employees commonly feel that the hearing protection impairs communication and therefore do not wear the hearing protection, or wear it incorrectly to increase their hearing capacity. On the basis of noise level measurements, hearing protection with a noise reduction rating of 15–20 dB would provide adequate protection even after adjusting for workplace conditions (i.e , subtracting 7 dB from the manufacturer's noise reduction rating and multiplying the result by 50%). Until TWA noise exposures for pharmacy technicians at the Baker machine are reduced below the OSHA AL and NIOSH REL, these employees should wear hearing protection, and a hearing conservation program should be implemented.

Many employees wore an earphone from a personal music player in one of their ears for much of the workday. Although the measured TWA noise exposures, with the exception of noise exposures near the Baker machine, should not present hearing loss risk, if the sound level from the earphone is greater than the background noise in the facility, employees could be at risk for hearing loss.

CONCLUSIONS

The airborne dust levels measured in the PBZs of employees at the mail order pharmacy contained APIs. We did not quantify exposures to all the APIs that were identified in air, but for those two that we did, exposures were below their applicable OELs. Using real-time particle meters, we identified releases of pharmaceutical dust during specific tasks, in particular the cleaning of cells and replenishment of canisters with tablets. Employees were exposed to APIs that they were not prescribed, which could be particularly harmful for individuals who are allergic to a particular API or taking medications that could interact

CONCLUSIONS (CONTINUED)

with low concentrations of APIs. However, allergic reactions and upper respiratory irritation are the most likely health effects from exposure to low levels of APIs. Most TWA noise exposures were below OSHA and NIOSH exposure limits. However, TWA noise exposures at the Baker machine can exceed the OSHA AL and NIOSH REL. The recommendations listed below will help minimize exposures to pharmaceutical dust and reduce noise levels.

RECOMMENDATIONS

Our recommendations are based on the hierarchy of controls approach (see Appendix B for more information). This approach groups actions by their likely effectiveness in reducing or removing hazards. In most cases, the preferred approach is to eliminate hazardous materials or processes and install engineering controls to reduce exposure or shield employees. Until such control measures are in place and shown to be effective, administrative controls or personal protective equipment may be needed. We encourage the pharmacy to use a labor-management health and safety committee or working group to discuss the recommendations in this report and develop an action plan.

Elimination and Substitution

Elimination or substitution of a hazardous process material is a highly effective means for reducing exposures. This strategy is most effective because it reduces the need for additional control measures in the future. However, we recognize that the elimination or substitution of materials is not always feasible.

1. Substitute uncoated tablets with coated tablets that are less likely to generate dust when choosing between uncoated and coated tablets that are pharmacologically the same.

Engineering Controls

Engineering controls reduce exposures to employees by removing the hazard from the process or placing a barrier between the hazard and the employee. Engineering controls are very effective at protecting employees without placing primary responsibility of implementation on the employee.

1. Install tabletop ventilation booths near the Baker and Optifill machines for use during the cleaning, repairing, and replenishment of Baker cells and Optifill canisters and in the hazardous drug area for use during the filling of hazardous drug prescriptions. Booths similar in design to a small tabletop paint booth would work well for this application. Figure VS-75-02 in "Industrial Ventilation: a Manual of Recommended Practice for Design" [ACGIH 2007], provides a design plan for this type of booth. Crossdraft ventilation is used for this type of booth to draw particles away from the product (and employees) and into particulate filters at the back of the booth. Position the booths at heights that minimize bending over or excessive reaching. Install a bracket in the ventilation booth for the Baker machine for holding the cells in an upright position during refilling.

2. Install movable capture hoods in the offline replenishment area for use during the replenishment of Baker canisters. Hoods similar in design to a capturing hood for low toxicity welding may work well for this application. Figure VS-90-02 in "Industrial Ventilation: a Manual of Recommended Practice for Design" [ACGIH 2007], provides a design plan for this type of hood. Instruct employees to place the inlet of the hoods near where dust is generated without interfering with the process. Install particulate filters on the negative pressure side of the exhaust fan.

3. Consult a ventilation specialist to design and install the booths and hoods and certify the booths annually.

4. Train employees annually on how to properly use and maintain the booths and hoods.

5. Reduce noise levels through the following noise controls:

   a. Install mufflers on the exhaust ports of solenoid valves and actuators, and investigate whether the air pressure in the compressed air system can be reduced.

   b. Maintain the compressed air system properly, and promptly repair leaks.

   c. At the capper, add a bottom panel, seal the gaps along the corners, and reduce the size of any openings.

   d. Reduce air pressure at the Optifill machine, and install a thicker plastic cover.

e. Install vibration isolation pads on equipment that generates low frequency noise near the capper, offline replenishment, and pharmacy station.

Administrative Controls

Administrative controls are management-dictated work practices and policies to reduce or prevent exposures to workplace hazards. The effectiveness of these control measures is dependent on management commitment and employee acceptance. Regular monitoring and reinforcement are necessary to ensure that following policies and procedures are not circumvented in the name of convenience or production.

1. Identify and label all hazardous drugs so that any employee can easily identify them [NIOSH 2010a].

2. Evaluate the potential for employee exposures from the dispensing of hazardous drugs in the automatic dispensing machines (estrogen). If these drugs can produce dust containing APIs during dispensing, then they should be transferred to the hazardous drug area where employee exposures can be more tightly controlled (see the next recommendation).

3. Modify standard operating procedures for the filling of hazardous drug prescriptions. The NIOSH Alert, "Preventing Occupational Exposure to Antineoplastic and Other Hazardous Drugs in Health Care Settings," provides guidelines on the control measures that should be used when handling hazardous drugs. These guidelines are intended primarily for oncology clinics and hospital pharmacies, but can be adapted for this mail order pharmacy. These procedures should include using a tabletop ventilation booth when filling hazardous drug prescriptions, wearing at least one pair of nitrile gloves, wearing a lab coat, and training employees on how to remove and discard gloves and clean the workstation so their skin is not contaminated. NIOSH-approved particulate respirators should be worn until the ventilation booth or other local exhaust ventilation system is available to use (see personal protective equipment recommendations).

4. Develop written standard operating procedures and a schedule for the change out of particulate filters used in the ventilation booths, hoods, and HEPA vacuums. These filters

could expose employees to pharmaceutical dust (including hazardous drugs) if proper safeguards are not in place. These procedures should involve a team of two employees who wear disposable gloves, disposable gowns, safety glasses, and NIOSH-approved particulate respirators (see personal protective equipment recommendations). One employee should hold a plastic bag, while the other employee removes the filter and places it in the bag. The bag should then be sealed. A HEPA vacuum should be used to collect any residual dust on surfaces. After replacing the filters, all PPE should be sealed in a plastic bag for disposal.

5. Use the HEPA vacuum daily to collect pharmaceutical dust that accumulates under the Baker cell nozzles, Optifill canisters, and other areas where pharmaceutical dust may collect.

6. Provide easier access to hand washing stations, and continue to require employees to wash their hands before eating or using tobacco products to prevent the hand-to-mouth ingestion of pharmaceutical particles.

7. Ensure that employees are not using compressed air for cleaning cells. Remove the compressed airline and nozzle if it is no longer needed.

8. Have employees report any workplace symptoms to their supervisors, who may in turn refer them for medical evaluation as appropriate.

9. Organize a health and safety committee consisting of employee and management representatives who meet regularly to address health and safety concerns.

10. Eliminate the use of personal music players in work areas.

11. Implement a hearing conservation program if noise exposures at the Baker machine cannot be reduced below the OSHA AL.

Personal Protective Equipment

PPE is the least effective means for controlling employee exposures. Proper use of PPE requires a comprehensive program, and calls for a high level of employee involvement and commitment to be effective. The use of PPE requires the selection of the appropriate equipment to reduce the hazard and the development of supporting programs such as training, change-out schedules, and

Recommendations (CONTINUED)

medical assessment if needed. PPE should not be relied upon as the sole method for limiting employee exposures. Rather, PPE should be used until engineering and administrative controls reduce exposures to acceptable levels.

1. Require employees to wear NIOSH-approved half-mask N95 filtering facepiece respirators or other NIOSH-approved particulate respirators with comparable or higher protection factors during the hand filling of hazardous drug prescriptions and change-out of particulate filters in the ventilation booths, hoods, and HEPA vacuums. Discontinue the use of respirators for hand filling hazardous drug prescriptions once a ventilation booth or other local exhaust ventilation system is available for this process and demonstrated to be effective in limiting dust exposures. Include employees required to wear respirators in a comprehensive respiratory protection program that adheres to the OSHA standard [29 CFR 1910.134].

2. Provide employees with lab coats or other personal protective clothing that can be discarded after use or laundered weekly by professionals. This will help prevent the contamination of personal clothing with APIs and minimize secondary exposures.

3. Emphasize to employees the importance of wearing nitrile gloves when handling pharmaceuticals.

4. Provide hearing protection with a noise reduction rating of 15–20 dB, and require that pharmacy technicians working around the Baker machine use the hearing protection.

References

ACGIH [2001]. Warfarin. In: Documentation of the threshold limit values and biological exposure indices. Cincinnati, OH: American Conference of Governmental Industrial Hygienists.

ACGIH [2007]. Industrial ventilation: a manual of recommended practice for design, 26th edition. Cincinnati, OH: American Conference of Governmental Industrial Hygienists.

ACGIH [2011]. Threshold limit values for chemical substances and physical agents and biological exposure indices. Cincinnati, OH: American Conference of Governmental Industrial Hygienists.

REFERENCES
(CONTINUED)

Brent RL, Tanski S, Weitzman M [2004]. A pediatric perspective on the unique vulnerability and resilience of the embryo and the child to environmental toxicants: the importance of rigorous research concerning age and agent. Pediatrics 113(4 Suppl):935–944.

Bristol-Myers Squibb Company [2008]. Safety data sheet: Lisinopril. [http://www.bmsmsds.com/msdsweb/filebrowse?objectid=0900dfd480336149]. Date accessed: October 2011.

CFR. Code of Federal Regulations. Washington, DC: U.S. Government Printing Office, Office of the Federal Register.

Hinds WC [1999]. Respiratory deposition. In: Aerosol technology: properties, behavior, and measurement of airborne particles. New York: John Wiley & Sons, Inc.

Hornung RW, Reed LD [1990]. Estimation of average concentration in the presence of non-detectable values. Appl Occup Environ Hyg 5(1):46–51.

Kenny LC, Aitken R, Chalmers C, Fabries JF, Gonzalez-Fernandez E, Kromhout H, Liden G, Mark D, Riediger G, Prodi V [1997]. A collaborative European study of personal inhalable aerosol sampler performance. Ann Occup Hyg 41(2):135–153.

NIOSH [2004]. NIOSH alert: preventing occupational exposure to antineoplastic and other hazardous drugs in health care settings. Cincinnati, OH: U.S. Department of Health and Human Services, Centers for Disease Control, National Institute for Occupational Safety and Health, DHHS (NIOSH) Publication No. 2004-165.

NIOSH [2010a]. NIOSH list of antineoplastic and other hazardous drugs in health care settings 2010. Cincinnati, OH: U.S. Department of Health and Human Services, Centers for Disease Control, National Institute for Occupational Safety and Health, DHHS (NIOSH) Publication No. 2010-167.

NIOSH [2010b]. NIOSH pocket guide to chemical hazards. Cincinnati, OH: U.S. Department of Health and Human Services, Centers for Disease Control and Prevention, National Institute for Occupational Safety and Health (NIOSH) Publication No. 2010-168c. [http://www.cdc.gov/niosh/npg/]. Date accessed: October 2011.

NIOSH [2011]. NIOSH manual of analytical methods. 4th ed. Schlecht PC, O'Connor PF, eds. Cincinnati, OH: U.S. Department of Health and Human Services, Centers for Disease Control and Prevention, National Institute for Occupational Safety and Health, DHHS (NIOSH) Publication No. 94-113 (August 1994); 1st Supplement Publication 96-135, 2nd Supplement Publication 98-119, 3rd Supplement Publication 2003-154. [http://www.cdc.gov/niosh/docs/2003-154/].

Takats Z, Wiseman JM, Gologan B, Cooks RG [2004]. Mass spectrometry sampling under ambient conditions with desorption electrospray ionization. Science 306(5695):471–473.

APPENDIX A: ADDITIONAL INFORMATION ON SAMPLING AND ANALYTICAL METHODS

Air Sampling Methods

AirChek XR5000 pumps (SKC, Inc., Eighty Four, Pennsylvania) were calibrated for an airflow rate of 4 Lpm, and SKC AirChek 2000 pumps were calibrated for all other airflow rates listed in Table 1 (on page 6). All pumps were precalibrated and postcalibrated with the sample media connected. The respirable dust sampling train consisted of a metal cyclone (model GK 2.05, BGI, Inc., Waltham, Massachusetts) connected to a Personal DataRAM aerosol monitor (Thermo, Smyrna, Georgia). Air was drawn through the inlet of Tygon® tubing positioned in the employee's PBZ. According to guidelines from Thermo, use of the Tygon tubing should result in less than a 10% loss in particles smaller than 4 µm in diameter [Thermo 1995].

During both visits, we used a Met One HHPC-6 handheld airborne particle counter (Hach® Ultra Analytics, Inc., Loveland, Colorado) to identify releases of pharmaceutical dust into the air. During the first visit, we sampled approximately 0.5–1 liters of air with the particle counter before, during, and after specific tasks. During the second visit, we sampled 1 liter of air continuously (about every 30 seconds) throughout the workday. Spikes in particle counts suggested releases of pharmaceutical dust, which we were able to correlate with tasks involving specific APIs.

Analytical Methods

We used NIOSH analytical methods to measure total dust (NIOSH Method 0500), respirable dust (NIOSH Method 0600), and warfarin (NIOSH Method 5002) [NIOSH 2011]. The analytical method used by Prosolia to identify APIs on the surface of filters is described in the scientific literature [Takats et al. 2004].

The analytical methods used for the quantitation of lactose and lisinopril were internal methods developed by BVNA. These methods are briefly described below.

Lactose

Filters were removed from the IOM samplers and extracted in glass vials using 1 mL of deionized water. The samples were capped and swirled. After extraction, the samples were transferred to autosampler vials and analyzed by high performance liquid chromatography using the parameters below.

  Instrument: Dionex 3000
  Column: Dionex CarboPac PA1, 4 × 250 mm
  Column flow rate: 1 mL per minute
  Column temperature: Ambient
  Injection volume: 200 microliter
  Detector: Electrochemical detector
  Mobile phase: Isocratic, 200 millimolar sodium hydroxide in deionized water

Lisinopril

Filters were previously processed for quantitation of lactose and were already desorbed in 1 mL of deionized water. Samples were transferred to autosampler vials and analyzed by high performance liquid chromatography using the parameters below.

Instrument: Waters 2690 separations module

Column: Agilent Zorbax Bonus-RP, 5 μm column 250 × 4.6 mm

Column flow rate: 1 mL per minute

Column temperature: Ambient

Injection volume: 25 microliter

Detector: Waters 2487 dual wavelength ultraviolet detector

Wavelength: 210 nanometers

Run time: 12 minutes

Mobile phase: 85% buffer/15% acetonitrile (buffer=1000 mL deionized water/8.25mL triethanolamine/11.75 mL phosphoric acid)

Noise Sampling Methods

We used Larson-Davis (Provo, Utah) Spark® model 705P or model 706-RC noise dosimeters. Both models of dosimeters functioned identically. For employee monitoring, we attached the noise dosimeters to the employees' belts and fastened the small dosimeter microphones to the employees' shirts at a point midway between the ear and the outside of the shoulder. We placed one area monitor on top of a pharmacist desk near the Baker machine and two area monitors in the offline replenishment area. The area monitors were intended to represent exposures of an employee working in those areas for an entire work shift. We placed windscreens over the microphones during measurements to reduce or eliminate artifact noise that can occur if objects bump against an unprotected microphone.

The dosimeters collected noise data using three different settings so that we could directly compare the noise measurement results with the three different noise exposure limits referenced in this HHE report: the OSHA PEL, OSHA AL, and the NIOSH REL. OSHA uses a 90-dBA criterion and a 5-dB exchange rate for both the PEL and AL. However, the PEL has a 90-dBA threshold, and the AL has an 80-dBA threshold. NIOSH has an 85-dBA criterion and uses an 80-dBA threshold. During noise dosimetry measurements, noise levels below the threshold level are not integrated by the dosimeter for accumulation of dose and calculation of TWA noise level. The dosimeters averaged noise levels every second during monitoring. At the end of the work shift, the dosimeters were removed, and the noise measurement information stored in the dosimeters was downloaded to a computer for interpretation with Larson Davis Blaze® computer software. The dosimeters were calibrated before and after the measurement periods according to the manufacturer's instructions.

The sound level meters were equipped with 0.5-inch random incidence Type 1 electret microphones. The sound level meters were calibrated according to the manufacturer's instructions. Sound level meters were either handheld or mounted on a tripod at a height of approximately 5 feet.

References

NIOSH [2011]. NIOSH manual of analytical methods. 4th ed. Schlecht PC, O'Connor PF, eds. Cincinnati, OH: U.S. Department of Health and Human Services, Centers for Disease Control and Prevention, National Institute for Occupational Safety and Health, DHHS (NIOSH) Publication No. 94-113 (August 1994); 1st Supplement Publication 96-135, 2nd Supplement Publication 98-119, 3rd Supplement Publication 2003-154. [http://www.cdc.gov/niosh/docs/2003-154/].

Takats Z, Wiseman JM, Gologan B, Cooks RG [2004]. Mass spectrometry sampling under ambient conditions with desorption electrospray ionization. Science 306(5695):471–473.

Thermo [1995]. Thermo technical guidelines: Inlet tubing guidelines for MIE dust monitors. Franklin, MA: Thermo Electron Corporation Publication No. 19-A.

In evaluating the hazards posed by workplace exposures, NIOSH investigators use both mandatory (legally enforceable) and recommended OELs for chemical, physical, and biological agents as a guide for making recommendations. OELs have been developed by federal agencies and safety and health organizations to prevent the occurrence of adverse health effects from workplace exposures. Generally, OELs suggest levels of exposure that most employees may be exposed to for up to 10 hours per day, 40 hours per week, for a working lifetime, without experiencing adverse health effects. However, not all employees will be protected from adverse health effects even if their exposures are maintained below these levels. A small percentage may experience adverse health effects because of individual susceptibility, a preexisting medical condition, and/or a hypersensitivity (allergy). In addition, some hazardous substances may act in combination with other workplace exposures, the general environment, or with medications or personal habits of the employee to produce adverse health effects even if the occupational exposures are controlled at the level set by the exposure limit. Also, some substances can be absorbed by direct contact with the skin and mucous membranes in addition to being inhaled, which contributes to the individual's overall exposure.

Most OELs are expressed as a TWA exposure. A TWA refers to the average exposure during a normal 8- to 10-hour workday. Some chemical substances and physical agents have recommended STEL or ceiling values where adverse health effects are caused by exposures over a short period. Unless otherwise noted, the STEL is a 15-minute TWA exposure that should not be exceeded at any time during a workday, and the ceiling limit is an exposure that should not be exceeded at any time.

In the United States, OELs have been established by federal agencies, professional organizations, state and local governments, and other entities. Some OELs are legally enforceable limits, while others are recommendations. The U.S. Department of Labor OSHA PELs (29 CFR 1910 [general industry]; 29 CFR 1926 [construction industry]; and 29 CFR 1917 [maritime industry]) are legal limits enforceable in workplaces covered under the Occupational Safety and Health Act of 1970. NIOSH RELs are recommendations based on a critical review of the scientific and technical information available on a given hazard and the adequacy of methods to identify and control the hazard. NIOSH RELs can be found in the *NIOSH Pocket Guide to Chemical Hazards* [NIOSH 2010]. NIOSH also recommends different types of risk management practices (e.g., engineering controls, safe work practices, employee education/ training, personal protective equipment, and exposure and medical monitoring) to minimize the risk of exposure and adverse health effects from these hazards. Other OELs that are commonly used and cited in the United States include the TLVs recommended by ACGIH, a professional organization, and the WEELs recommended by the American Industrial Hygiene Association, another professional organization. The TLVs and WEELs are developed by committee members of these associations from a review of the published, peer-reviewed literature. They are not consensus standards. ACGIH TLVs are considered voluntary exposure guidelines for use by industrial hygienists and others trained in this discipline "to assist in the control of health hazards" [ACGIH 2011]. WEELs have been established for some chemicals "when no other legal or authoritative limits exist" [AIHA 2011].

Outside the United States, OELs have been established by various agencies and organizations and include both legal and recommended limits. The Institut für Arbeitsschutz der Deutschen Gesetzlichen Unfallversicherung (IFA, Institute for Occupational Safety and Health of the German Social Accident

Insurance) maintains a database of international OELs from European Union member states, Canada (Québec), Japan, Switzerland, and the United States. The database, available at http://www.dguv.de/ifa/en/gestis/limit_values/index.jsp, contains international limits for over 1,500 hazardous substances and is updated periodically.

Employers should understand that not all hazardous chemicals have specific OSHA PELs, and for some agents the legally enforceable and recommended limits may not reflect current health-based information. However, an employer is still required by OSHA to protect its employees from hazards even in the absence of a specific OSHA PEL. OSHA requires an employer to furnish employees a place of employment free from recognized hazards that cause or are likely to cause death or serious physical harm [Occupational Safety and Health Act of 1970 (Public Law 91–596, sec. 5(a)(1))]. Thus, NIOSH investigators encourage employers to make use of other OELs when making risk assessments and risk management decisions to best protect the health of their employees. NIOSH investigators also encourage the use of the traditional hierarchy of controls approach to eliminate or minimize identified workplace hazards. This includes, in order of preference, the use of (1) substitution or elimination of the hazardous agent, (2) engineering controls (e.g , local exhaust ventilation, process enclosure, dilution ventilation), (3) administrative controls (e.g., limiting time of exposure, employee training, work practice changes, medical surveillance), and (4) personal protective equipment (e.g., respiratory protection, gloves, eye protection, hearing protection). Control banding, a qualitative risk assessment and risk management tool, is a complementary approach to protecting employee health that focuses resources on exposure controls by describing how a risk needs to be managed. Information on control banding is available at http://www.cdc.gov/niosh/topics/ctrlbanding/. This approach can be applied in situations where OELs have not been established or can be used to supplement the OELs, when available.

Active Pharmaceutical Ingredients

Of the compounds we identified in air, only warfarin has an OEL established by a U.S. national agency or organization. Warfarin is an anticoagulant prescribed for people with certain types of irregular heartbeat, people with prosthetic (replacement or mechanical) heart valves, and people who have suffered a heart attack. Warfarin is also used to treat or prevent venous thrombosis (swelling and blood clot in a vein) and pulmonary embolism (a blood clot in the lung) [PubMed Health 2011]. The NIOSH REL, OSHA PEL, and ACGIH TLV for warfarin ($100 \ \mu g/m^3$) are based on the potential for hemorrhage of biological tissues [ACGIH 2001, NIOSH 2010]. ACGIH specifically states that its TLV is intended to minimize the potential for hemorrhage of the mucous membranes and gastrointestinal and genitourinary tracts [ACGIH 2001]. For the other APIs that we identified in air, Table B1 provides a summary of their therapeutic uses and manufacturers' OELs (if available). The manufacturers' OELs were established by pharmaceutical companies using a control banding process, which places APIs into hazard categories using data such as potency, severity of acute effects, lethal dose, irritation, and sensitization [Naumann et al. 1996; Naumann 2005; Zalk and Nelson 2008]. Hazard categories have acceptable levels of exposure or OELs.

Table B1. Prescribed uses and manufacturers' OELs for the APIs identified in air

API	Prescribed for*	Manufacturer OEL (µg/m³)†
Allopurinol	Gout	5,000
Benazepril	High blood pressure	None published
Bethanechol chloride	Urination problems	None published
Buspirone HCl	Anxiety	None published
Carbidopa / levodopa	Parkinson disease and Parkinson-like symptoms	100
Chlorpheniramine maleate	Allergies	10
Doxazosin mesylate	Enlarged prostate or high blood pressure	30
Glipizide	Type 2 diabetes	None published
Hydralazine HCl	High blood pressure	None published
Lamotrigine	Epileptic seizures, depression, mania and other abnormal moods in patients with bipolar disorder	200
Lisinopril	High blood pressure, heart failure	10
Meclizine HCl	Motion sickness	70
Metformin	Type 2 diabetes	800
Methocarbamol	Muscle pain	None published
Metoclopramide HCl	Heart burn, ulcers, acid reflux	40
Naproxen sodium	Pain, reducing fever	1,000
Oxybutynin	Overactive bladder	None published
Promethazine HCl	Allergies, conjunctivitis, skin reactions, motion sickness	None published
Sotalol HCl	Irregular heartbeat	None published
Trazadone HCl	Depression	None published
Venlafaxine HCl	Depression, anxiety, panic disorder	250

* [PubMed Health 2011]

† Allopurinol [GlaxoSmithKline 2006], carbidopa [Bristol-Myers Squibb Company 2010], chlorpheniramine maleate [GlaxoSmithKline 2005], doxazosin mesylate [Pfizer 2009], lamotrigine [GlaxoSmithKline 2007], lisinopril [Bristol-Myers Squibb Company 2008a], meclizine HCl [Pfizer 2003], metformin [Bristol-Myers Squibb Company 2008b], metoclopramide HCl [Hospira 2008], naproxen sodium [Roche 2006], venlafaxine [Pfizer 2007]

Appendix B: Occupational Exposure Limits and Health Effects (continued)

Noise

Noise-induced hearing loss is an irreversible, sensorineural condition that progresses with exposure. Although hearing ability declines with age (presbycusis), noise exposure produces more hearing loss than that resulting from aging alone. This noise-induced hearing loss is caused by damage to nerve cells of the inner ear (cochlea) and, unlike some conductive hearing disorders, cannot be treated medically [Berger et al. 2003]. In most cases, noise-induced hearing loss develops slowly and usually occurs before it is noticed. Hearing loss is often severe enough to permanently affect a person's ability to hear and understand speech. For example, people with hearing loss may not be able to distinguish words such as "fish" from "fist" [Suter 1978].

The dBA is the preferred unit for measuring sound levels to assess employee noise exposures. The dBA noise scale is weighted to approximate the sensory response of human ears to sound frequencies near the hearing threshold. Because the dBA scale is logarithmic, increases of 3 dBA, 10 dBA, and 20 dBA represent a doubling, tenfold increase, and hundredfold increase of sound energy, respectively. Noise exposures expressed in dBA cannot be averaged by taking the arithmetic mean.

The OSHA noise standard [29 CFR 1910.95] specifies a PEL of 90 dBA, as an 8-hour TWA. The OSHA PEL is calculated using a 5-dB exchange rate. This means that a person may be exposed to noise levels of 95 dBA for no more than 4 hours, 100 dBA for 2 hours, 105 dBA for 1 hour, etc. An employee's daily noise dose, based on the duration and intensity of noise exposure, can be calculated according to the formula

$$\text{Dose} = 100 \times (C_1/T_1 + C_2/T_2 + \ldots + C_n/T_n),$$

where C_n indicates the total time of exposure at a specific noise level and T_n indicates the reference duration for that level as given in Table G-16a of the OSHA noise regulation. Doses greater than 100% are in excess of the OSHA PEL.

When noise exposures exceed the PEL of 90 dBA, OSHA requires that employees wear hearing protection, and that an employer implement feasible engineering or administrative controls to reduce noise exposures. The OSHA noise standard also requires an employer to implement a hearing conservation program when 8-hour TWA noise exposures exceed the AL 85 dBA. The program must include noise monitoring, employee notification, observation, audiometric testing, hearing protectors, training, and record keeping.

NIOSH [NIOSH 1998] and ACGIH [ACGIH 2011] recommend an exposure limit of 85 dBA, as an 8-hour TWA. A more conservative 3 dB exchange rate is used in calculating exposure these limits. Using NIOSH criteria, an employee can be exposed to 85 dBA for 8 hours, but to no more than 88 dBA for 4 hours, 91 dBA for 2 hours, 94 dBA for 1 hour, etc. Twelve-hour exposures have to be 83.2 dBA or less according to the NIOSH REL.

Audiometric evaluations of employees hearing thresholds must be conducted in quiet locations, preferably in a sound-attenuating booth, by presenting pure tones of varying frequencies at threshold levels (i.e , the level of a sound that the person can just barely hear). Zero dB hearing level represents the hearing level of an average, young individual with good hearing. OSHA requires hearing thresholds to be measured at test frequencies of 500, 1,000, 2,000, 3,000, 4,000, and 6,000 Hz. Individual employee's annual audiograms are compared to their baseline audiogram to determine if a standard threshold shift has occurred. OSHA states that a standard threshold shift has occurred if the average threshold values at 2,000, 3,000, and 4,000 Hz have increased by 10 dB or more in either ear when comparing the annual audiogram to the baseline audiogram [29 CFR 1910.95]. The NIOSH-recommended hearing threshold shift criterion is a 15-dB shift at any frequency in either ear from 500–6,000 Hz measured twice in succession [NIOSH 1998]. Both of these hearing threshold shift criteria require at least two audiometric tests.

The audiogram profile is a plot of the hearing test frequencies (x-axis) versus the hearing threshold levels (y-axis). For many employees, the audiogram profile tends to slope downward toward the high frequencies with an improvement at the audiogram's highest frequencies, forming a "notch" [Suter 2002]. A notch in the audiogram of an employee with otherwise normal hearing may indicate the early onset of hearing loss. The notch from occupational noise can occur between 3,000 and 6,000 Hz [ACOM 1989; Osguthorpe and Klein 2001]. However, it is generally accepted that a notch at 4,000 Hz indicates occupational hearing loss [Prince et al. 1997]. An individual may have notches at different frequencies in one or both ears [Suter 2002]. For this evaluation, a notch is defined as the frequency where the hearing level is preceded by an improvement of at least 10 dB and followed by an improvement of at least 5 dB.

References

ACGIH [2001]. Warfarin. In: Documentation of the threshold limit values and biological exposure indices. Cincinnati, OH: American Conference of Governmental Industrial Hygienists.

ACGIH [2011]. Threshold limit values for chemical substances and physical agents and biological exposure indices. Cincinnati, OH: American Conference of Governmental Industrial Hygienists.

ACOM [1989]. Occupational noise-induced hearing loss. ACOM Noise and Hearing Conservation Committee. J Occup Med 31(12):996.

AIHA [2011]. AIHA 2009 Emergency response planning guidelines (ERPG) & workplace environmental exposure levels (WEEL) handbook. Fairfax, VA: American Industrial Hygiene Association.

Berger EH, Royster LH, Royster JD, Driscoll DP, Layne M, eds. [2003]. The noise manual. 5th rev. ed. Fairfax, VA: American Industrial Hygiene Association.

Bristol-Myers Squibb Company [2008a]. Safety data sheet: Lisinopril. [http://www.bmsmsds.com/msdsweb/filebrowse?objectid=0900dfd480336149]. Date accessed: September 2011.

Bristol-Myers Squibb Company [2008b]. Safety data sheet: Metformin hydrochloride. [http://www.bmsmsds.com/msdsweb/filebrowse?objectid=0900dfd480335b4f]. Date accessed: September 2011.

Bristol-Myers Squibb Company [2010]. Safety data sheet: Sinemet tablets - bulk and drug product. [http://www.bmsmsds.com/msdsweb/filebrowse?objectid=0900dfd48038c302]. Date accessed: September 2011.

CFR. Code of Federal Regulations. Washington, DC: U.S. Government Printing Office, Office of the Federal Register.

GlaxoSmithKline [2005]. Safety data sheet: Piriton syrup. [http://www.msds-gsk.com/uk_cons/12732103.pdf]. Date accessed: September 2011.

GlaxoSmithKline [2006]. Safety data sheet: Zyloric tablets. [http://www.msds-gsk.com/uk_presc/12703205.pdf]. Date accessed: September 2011.

GlaxoSmithKline [2007]. Safety data sheet: Lamictal dispersible tablets. [http://www.msds-gsk.com/12701905.pdf]. Date accessed: September 2011.

Hospira [2008]. Safety data sheet: Metoclopramide. [http://www.bdipharma.com/MSDS/Hospira/Metoclopramide.pdf]. Date accessed: September 2011.

Naumann BD [2005]. Control banding in the pharmaceutical industry. [http://www.aioh.org.au/downloads/documents/ControlBandingBNaumann.pdf]. Date accessed: September 2011.

Naumann BD, Sargent EV, Starkman BS, Fraser WJ, Becker GT, Kirk GD [1996]. Performance-based exposure control limits for pharmaceutical active ingredients. Am Ind Hyg Assoc J 57(1):33–42.

NIOSH [1998]. Criteria for a recommended standard: Occupational noise exposure (revised criteria 1998). Cincinnati, OH: U.S. Department of Health and Human Services, Centers for Disease Control and Prevention, National Institute for Occupational Safety and Health, DHHS (NIOSH) Publication No. 98-126.

NIOSH [2010]. NIOSH pocket guide to chemical hazards. Cincinnati, OH: U.S. Department of Health and Human Services, Centers for Disease Control and Prevention, National Institute for Occupational Safety and Health (NIOSH) Publication No. 2010-168c. [http://www.cdc.gov/niosh/npg/]. Date accessed: October 2011.

NIOSH [2010]. NIOSH list of antineoplastic and other hazardous drugs in health care settings 2010. Cincinnati, OH: U.S. Department of Health and Human Services, Centers for Disease Control, National Institute for Occupational Safety and Health, DHHS (NIOSH) Publication No. 2010-167.

Osguthorpe JD, Klein AJ [2001]. Occupational hearing conservation. Clinical Audiology 24(2):403–414.

Pfizer [2003]. Safety data sheet: Antivert (meclizine hydrochloride) tablets. [http://www.pfizer.com/files/products/material_safety_data/193.pdf]. Date accessed: September 2011.

Pfizer [2007]. Safety data sheet: Effexor products. [http://www.pfizer.com/files/products/material_safety_data/WP00005.pdf]. Date accessed: September 2011.

Pfizer [2009]. Safety data sheet: Doxazosin mesylate. [http://www.pfizer.com/files/products/material_safety_data/PZ01040.pdf]. Date accessed: September 2011.

Prince M, Stayner L, Smith R, Gilbert S [1997]. A re-examination of risk estimates from the NIOSH Occupational Noise and Hearing Survey (ONHS). J Acous Soc Am 101(2):950–963.

PubMed Health [2011]. Drugs and Supplements. [http://www.ncbi.nlm.nih.gov/pubmedhealth/s/drugs_and_supplements/a/]. Date accessed: September 2011.

Roche [2006]. Safety data sheet: Naproxen sodium. [http://www.roche.com/pages/csds/english/out/0490628.20110225.8049_pdf]. Date accessed: September 2011.

Suter AH [1978]. The ability of mildly-impaired individuals to discriminate speech in noise. Washington, DC: U.S. Environmental Protection Agency, Joint EPA/USAF study, EPA 550/9-78-100, AMRL-TR-78-4.

Suter AH [2002]. Hearing conservation manual. 4th ed. Milwaukee, WI: Council for Accreditation in Occupational Hearing Conservation.

Zalk DM, Nelson DI [2008]. History and evolution of control banding: a review. J Occup Environ Hyg 5(5):330–346.

This page left intentionally blank

Acknowledgments and Availability of Report

The Hazard Evaluations and Technical Assistance Branch (HETAB) of the National Institute for Occupational Safety and Health (NIOSH) conducts field investigations of possible health hazards in the workplace. These investigations are conducted under the authority of Section 20(a)(6) of the Occupational Safety and Health Act of 1970, 29 U.S.C. 669(a)(6) which authorizes the Secretary of Health and Human Services, following a written request from any employer or authorized representative of employees, to determine whether any substance normally found in the place of employment has potentially toxic effects in such concentrations as used or found. HETAB also provides, upon request, technical and consultative assistance to federal, state, and local agencies; labor; industry; and other groups or individuals to control occupational health hazards and to prevent related trauma and disease.

Mention of any company or product does not constitute endorsement by NIOSH. In addition, citations to websites external to NIOSH do not constitute NIOSH endorsement of the sponsoring organizations or their programs or products. Furthermore, NIOSH is not responsible for the content of these websites. All Web addresses referenced in this document were accessible as of the publication date.

This report was prepared by Kenneth Fent, Srinivas Durgam, Carlos Aristeguieta, and Scott Brueck of HETAB, Division of Surveillance, Hazard Evaluations and Field Studies. Elena Page of HETAB assisted with the interpretation of the medical interview data and Donna Heidel of NIOSH Education and Information Division assisted with the interpretation of the active pharmaceutical ingredient exposure data. Industrial hygiene field assistance was provided by Chad Dowell and Diana Ceballos of HETAB. Industrial hygiene equipment and logistical support was provided by Donnie Booher and Karl Feldmann. Analytical support was provided by BVNA and Justin Wiseman and Joseph Kennedy at Prosolia, Indianapolis, Indiana. Health communication assistance was provided by Stefanie Evans. Editorial assistance was provided by Ellen Galloway. Desktop publishing was performed by Greg Hartle.

Copies of this report have been sent to employee and management representatives at the mail order pharmacy, the state health department, and the Occupational Safety and Health Administration Regional Office. This report is not copyrighted and may be freely reproduced. The report may be viewed and printed at http://www.cdc.gov/niosh/hhe/. Copies may be purchased from the National Technical Information Service at 5825 Port Royal Road, Springfield, Virginia 22161.

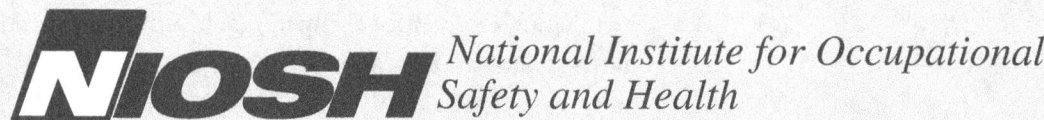

National Institute for Occupational Safety and Health

Delivering on the Nation's promise: Safety and health at work for all people through research and prevention.

To receive NIOSH documents or information about occupational safety and health topics, contact NIOSH at:

1-800-CDC-INFO (1-800-232-4636)

TTY: 1-888-232-6348

E-mail: cdcinfo@cdc.gov

or visit the NIOSH web site at: **www.cdc.gov/niosh**.

For a monthly update on news at NIOSH, subscribe to NIOSH eNews by visiting **www.cdc.gov/niosh/eNews**.

SAFER • HEALTHIER • PEOPLE™